T0368414

BOUNDARIES
A N D
BALANCE

GUIDE TO PROTECTING YOUR PEACE

LENISE "HARMONY" HALLEY MM. MDIV.

BALBOA.PRESS

A DIVISION OF HAY HOUSE

Balboa Press books may be ordered through booksellers or by contacting:

Balboa Press
A Division of Hay House
1663 Liberty Drive
Bloomington, IN 47403
www.balboapress.com
844-682-1282

Because of the dynamic nature of the Internet, any web addresses or
links contained in this book may have changed since publication and
may no longer be valid. The views expressed in this work are solely those
of the author and do not necessarily reflect the views of the publisher,
and the publisher hereby disclaims any responsibility for them.

The author of this book does not dispense medical advice or prescribe the use
of any technique as a form of treatment for physical, emotional, or medical
problems without the advice of a physician, either directly or indirectly. The
intent of the author is only to offer information of a general nature to help
you in your quest for emotional and spiritual well-being. In the event you use
any of the information in this book for yourself, which is your constitutional
right, the author and the publisher assume no responsibility for your actions.

Any people depicted in stock imagery provided by Getty Images are
models, and such images are being used for illustrative purposes only.
Certain stock imagery © Getty Images.

Print information available on the last page.

ISBN: 979-8-7652-5578-0 (sc)
ISBN: 979-8-7652-5577-3 (e)

Balboa Press rev. date: 12/11/2024

CONTENTS

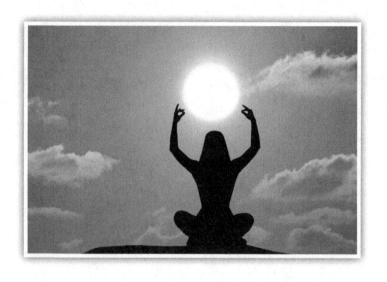

INTRODUCTION

As an International Coaching Federation Professional Certified Coach, Certified Personal Trainer, Reiki Master Teacher, and Yoga Teacher, I have guided individuals on transformative journeys toward holistic well-being. Throughout my career, I have witnessed firsthand the profound impact that setting boundaries can have on one's physical, emotional, and spiritual health. Drawing upon my diverse background and expertise in coaching, fitness, energy healing, yoga philosophy, and Reiki principles, I have developed a comprehensive approach to supporting individuals in establishing healthy boundaries that honor their unique needs and priorities.

Healthy boundaries may not be central to your upbringing, but they can be learned. Boundaries are about where you end and another person begins. Creating healthy boundaries takes patience, the ability to say "No," and clear communication to outline where the boundary lines are drawn. Some boundaries are social or cultural norms. Most of us are taught at a young age to give people space, keep our hands to ourselves, or understand that some things are not ours, so we start to understand boundaries as they are presented to us. I was taught as a child that when I entered a room, I was to greet the adults. We called before we went to someone's house and got permission before we passed someone's phone number along to someone else.

I learned not to call or attempt to go to my friend's house too early in the morning. I also only call people after 8:00 pm with their expressed wishes. You must take your shoes off in some households when entering the house. In other households, everyone eats at the table for dinner, or food is prohibited in different areas of the house. Some people do not like others to eat in their car. In all these examples, people generally clarify what someone should or should not do regarding their person or property. As we age, we must learn how to set boundaries for ourselves. I have found that boundaries and balance are made clear by observing our bodies' natural boundaries through the lens of the eight limbs of yoga and Reiki. These practices enhance our well-being and empower us to maintain healthier, more respectful relationships.

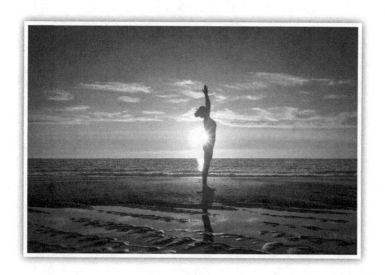

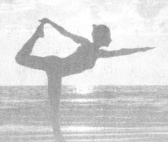

CHAPTER 1

Exploring Boundaries Inside and Outside the Body

The Breath Of The Body

There are many gems in the yoga philosophy; for the sake of brevity, I will only focus on the Eight Limbs, which provide a framework for living a balanced and harmonious life. Among these limbs is Pranayama, the practice of breath work, which emphasizes the importance of conscious breathing for nurturing our life force energy (prana) and promoting inner peace and clarity.

> *"When that [steadiness of posture] is acquired, breath control [Pranayama] follows, which is the regulation of the incoming and outgoing breath."* (Chapter 2, Sutra 49)

Similarly, in Reiki philosophy, we recognize the vital role of energy flow in maintaining health and well-being, and we learn techniques to channel and balance this energy for healing and transformation throughout the body.

We all know breathing is vital to our existence. As much as we understand it is critical, it is also very passive. We breathe without thinking. We only think about breathing when we cannot breathe passively. Breathing is as spiritually enriching as it is biologically necessary. No matter your cosmological belief, our breath is what gives us life. Our ability to breathe in oxygen and transport it through our body feeds life to our blood and travels through the rest of us. Breathing is rhythmic, restorative, and rejuvenating.

Our breathing changes when we are angry, anxious, scared, or triggered in other ways; we stop breathing or fail to breathe deeply enough for gas exchange to be effective, and we starve our bodies of life. We allow outside influences to damage our quality of life from the inside out. No matter your current state, re-centering on breathing is a significant step to living well. It seems simple, but it can be challenging. Simple can be difficult.

Conscious breathing is when we switch focus to our ability to inhale, hold our breath, and exhale. These three steps, done consciously, improve our ability and the quality of our breath. Let's start with the inhale. Sitting or standing straight, take a deep breath in. Imagine breathing in through your nose and into the bottom of your lungs. Hold your breath briefly, then blow out slowly. Try to clear all the air out before you start the process over. After you repeat the breathing process a few times, you can reason better. You have the mental space to process what is happening inside you. When you are triggered, or in any other way in a fight, flight, freeze, or fawn response, your prefrontal cortex turns off, and your amygdala takes over, prohibiting conscious rational thought. This response is part of the body's natural defense mechanism, designed to protect you from perceived threats.

The Prefrontal Cortex and Rational Thought: The prefrontal cortex, located at the front of the brain, is responsible for higher-order functions such as reasoning, decision-making, and self-control. It allows you to think logically, plan for the future, and regulate your emotions. The prefrontal cortex helps you assess situations calmly and respond with full rationality when functioning optimally.

The Amygdala and Survival Instincts: The amygdala, part of the limbic system, plays a crucial role in processing emotions, particularly fear and stress. It also acts as an alarm system, detecting potential threats and triggering the body's survival responses. When the amygdala perceives danger, it sends signals that activate the fight, flight, freeze, or fawn responses.

Fight, Flight, Freeze, or Fawn Response:

- Fight: Preparing to confront the threat aggressively.
- Flight: Readying to escape from the danger.
- Freeze: Becoming immobile, hoping the threat will pass unnoticed.
- Fawn: Attempting to appease or placate the danger.

These responses are automatic and instinctual, designed to ensure immediate survival. However, in modern life, these reactions can be triggered by non-life-threatening stressors, such as a heated argument, work pressure, or social anxiety.

Disconnection of the Prefrontal Cortex: During a fight, flight, freeze, or fawn response, the brain prioritizes survival over rational thinking. The amygdala hijacks the brain's resources, diverting blood flow and energy away from the prefrontal cortex to the more primitive parts of the brain. This process, known as amygdala hijack, results in:

- Impaired Decision-Making: Reduced ability to think clearly and make rational choices.
- Emotional Reactivity: Heightened emotions, making it difficult to control anger, fear, or anxiety.
- Loss of Perspective: Difficulty seeing the bigger picture or considering long-term consequences.

Reclaiming Rational Thought: Reclaiming access to the prefrontal cortex and restoring rational thinking are essential to calm the amygdala and deactivate the stress response. Techniques such as deep breathing, meditation, and grounding exercises can help shift the brain from a reactive state to a more balanced, reflective one. These techniques can enhance your ability to manage stress, set healthy boundaries, and respond to challenges comfortably.

Understanding the brain's response to stress underscores the importance of strategies that help regain control and clarity. Pranayama plays a crucial role in this process. When we are in a trauma response, such as fight, flight, freeze, or fawn, our prefrontal cortex shuts down, and our amygdala takes over. This shift inhibits rational thought and heightens emotional reactivity. Focusing on our breath—which can include breathwork, breath control, or energy control—can calm the amygdala and re-engage the prefrontal cortex, effectively moving out of a trauma response and into a state of calm and rationality.

The Human Body is a Complex System of Boundaries

The human body operates with a complex system of boundaries at various physical and energetic levels. These boundaries maintain the integrity and functionality of the body's systems, ensuring optimal health and well-being. Let's explore how the body physically operates with healthy boundaries:

Cellular Boundaries: At the cellular level, cell membranes act as boundaries that separate the cell's interior from its external environment. This semi-permeable membrane regulates the passage of substances in and out of the cell, allowing nutrients to enter while keeping harmful substances out. This selective permeability is crucial for cellular function and maintaining cellular homeostasis.

Tissue Boundaries: Different types of tissues in the body are organized into distinct layers or structures, each with its boundaries. These tissue boundaries provide structural support, protect internal organs, and facilitate cell communication. For example, the epidermis (outer layer of the skin) acts as a barrier that protects the body from external pathogens and regulates temperature and moisture levels.

Organ Boundaries: Organs within the body are enclosed within membranes or connective tissue layers that serve as boundaries separating them from surrounding tissues. These organ boundaries help maintain the structural integrity of organs, prevent them from shifting or collapsing, and facilitate their proper functioning. For example, the pericardium encloses the heart, providing protection and support while allowing for its rhythmic contractions.

Fluid Dynamics: The body contains various fluids, such as blood, lymph, cerebrospinal fluid, and interstitial fluid, which are crucial in transporting nutrients, removing waste products, regulating temperature, and maintaining homeostasis. Boundaries between these fluids ensure their proper compartmentalization and prevent mixing, which could disrupt their functions. For example, blood vessels act as boundaries that contain blood within specific circulatory pathways, ensuring its flow to vital organs while preventing leakage into surrounding tissues.

Energetic Boundaries: Besides physical boundaries, the body also has energetic boundaries that regulate the flow of subtle energy (such as prana in yoga or ki in Reiki) throughout the body. These energetic boundaries, often associated with the aura or energy field, help protect the body from external influences and maintain energetic balance. Practices like yoga, qigong, and Reiki aim to strengthen and balance these energetic boundaries to support overall health and well-being.

The body operates with healthy boundaries at multiple levels, from cellular membranes to organ structures, to ensure proper functioning and maintain homeostasis. These boundaries protect and support the body's various systems, facilitate communication and exchange of nutrients and waste products, and regulate the flow of fluids and energy. By understanding and nurturing these boundaries, individuals can promote optimal health and vitality in their physical and energetic bodies. In addition, by recognizing and respecting these natural boundaries, we can better understand how to apply similar principles to our interactions and relationships.

> *"By the practice of the different parts of yoga, impurities are destroyed; the crown of knowledge radiates in glory." (Patanjali, 2:28)*

Listening to Your Body: A Guide to Recognizing the Need for Boundaries

Your body is an incredibly intuitive and wise instrument, constantly sending signals and cues to alert you to its needs and boundaries. From subtle sensations to unmistakable physical sensations, your body provides valuable feedback that can guide you in recognizing when to set boundaries in your life.

Physical Sensations: Pay attention to bodily sensations such as tension, fatigue, or discomfort. These sensations often indicate that your boundaries are being violated or that you are expending more energy than you can sustain. Notice any changes in your posture, breathing patterns, or muscle tension, as these may reflect your body's response to stress or overwhelm.

Emotional Responses: Your emotions can be powerful indicators of when your boundaries have been crossed. Notice resentment, anger, or frustration, which may arise when your boundaries are disregarded, or you neglect to assert your needs. Be mindful of emotional shifts such as anxiety, sadness, or irritability, as these may signal that you need more excellent self-care and boundary-setting.

Intuitive Insights: Trust your intuition, which often communicates through subtle nudges, gut feelings, or intuitive hunches. Pay attention to any intuitive insights or inner guidance that prompt you to take action or make changes in your life. Tune into your inner wisdom, which may speak to you through dreams, synchronicities, or moments of clarity and inspiration.

Energy Levels: Your energy levels can provide valuable information about your overall well-being and the state of your boundaries. Notice fluctuations in your energy throughout the day, and pay attention to any patterns or trends. Be aware of times when you feel drained, depleted, or overwhelmed, as these may indicate that your boundaries need to be strengthened or reestablished.

Sensory Awareness: Engage your senses to deepen your awareness of your body and its boundaries. Notice sensations of touch, taste, smell, sight, and sound and how they impact your overall sense of comfort and safety. Use sensory grounding techniques—such as focusing on your breath, feeling the ground beneath your feet, or tuning into the natural world around you—to anchor yourself in the present moment and connect with your body's wisdom. By tuning into your body and listening to its signals, you can gain valuable insights into when it's time to set boundaries in your life. Trust yourself to honor your body's needs and prioritize your well-being, knowing that setting boundaries is an act of self-love and self-care that allows you to live authentically and thrive.

Understanding the importance of breath in the body and recognizing its role in regulating our stress response illuminates the natural boundaries our bodies have built to maintain health and balance. This awareness underscores why we turn to the philosophies of yoga and Reiki as guideposts for setting boundaries and achieving a healthy balance. Both practices are holistic modalities that emphasize inner peace and healing. By integrating the principles of pranayama and Reiki energy work, we can cultivate a deeper connection with ourselves, fostering an environment where healthy boundaries thrive promoting overall well-being and harmonious relationships.

Exploring Boundaries and Their Resonance with Personal Growth

Exploring boundaries and their resonance with personal growth involves exploring how establishing, maintaining, and respecting boundaries can foster individual development and well-being. Here's an expanded exploration of this concept:

Understanding Boundaries as Growth Opportunities:
Boundaries are not just limits we set to protect ourselves; they also serve as opportunities for personal growth. Reflecting on boundaries allows individuals to recognize the areas where they need to assert themselves, communicate their needs, and honor their values. By acknowledging these boundaries, individuals can embark on self-discovery and empowerment.

Identifying Patterns and Triggers: Exploring boundaries involves identifying recurring patterns and triggers that may indicate where boundaries are needed. This self-awareness allows individuals to understand why certain situations or relationships drain their energy or cause discomfort. By recognizing these patterns, individuals can explore underlying beliefs, fears, or past experiences that influence boundary-setting behavior.

Exploring Comfort Zones and Growth Edges: Boundaries often delineate the edges of our comfort zones, indicating where we feel safe and secure versus where we feel challenged or vulnerable. Reflecting on boundaries encourages individuals to explore their growth edges—the areas beyond their comfort zones where personal development occurs. By stretching these boundaries incrementally, individuals can expand their capacity for resilience, adaptability, and self-confidence.

Honoring Self-Care and Well-Being: Boundaries are essential for self-care and well-being. Exploring boundaries involves considering how honoring one's needs and limits improves overall health and happiness. It requires individuals to prioritize self-care practices, such as rest, relaxation, and stress management, and to recognize when they need to say no or set boundaries to protect their physical, emotional, and mental health.

Navigating Relationships and Interactions: Boundaries play a crucial role in navigating relationships and interactions with others. Reflecting on boundaries allows individuals to discern healthy from unhealthy dynamics, assert their autonomy and agency, and cultivate mutually respectful relationships. It involves communicating boundaries assertively and compassionately while also respecting others' boundaries.

Embracing Change and Evolution: Reflecting on boundaries acknowledges that boundaries are not fixed but evolve as individuals grow and change. It involves embracing the fluidity of boundaries and being open to reassessing and adjusting them as circumstances and needs shift. This flexibility allows individuals to adapt to new challenges, opportunities, and stages of life with greater ease and resilience.

Cultivating Empowerment and Authenticity: Ultimately, reflecting on boundaries empowers individuals to live authentically and align with their true selves. It involves embracing vulnerability, authenticity, and self-expression, even in the face of resistance or criticism. By honoring their boundaries, individuals cultivate a sense of agency, integrity, and wholeness, leading to greater fulfillment and personal growth.

In essence, exploring boundaries and their resonance with personal growth invites individuals to embark on a journey of self-discovery, empowerment, and authenticity. It encourages individuals to explore the edges of their comfort zones, honor their needs and values, and cultivate healthy relationships and lifestyles that support their well-being and evolution.

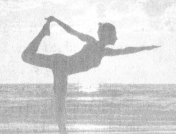

CHAPTER 2

Boundaries from Both Yogic and Reiki Perspectives

Boundaries play a crucial role in personal growth and well-being from both yogic and Reiki perspectives. Let's explore their significance.

From a Yogic Perspective

> *"Yoga teaches us to cure what need not be endured and endure what cannot be cured."*
> (B.K.S. Iyengar, *Light on Life*)

Maintaining Energetic Balance: In yoga philosophy, the human body is seen as a complex system of energy channels (nadis) and centers (chakras). Boundaries help regulate the flow of energy within this system, ensuring one's energy remains balanced and harmonious. Without clear boundaries, energy can become depleted or stagnant, leading to physical, emotional, and spiritual imbalances.

Honoring the Self: Yoga teaches the importance of self-awareness and self-care. Setting boundaries is an act of self-respect and self-love, affirming one's worth and prioritizing personal well-being. By establishing boundaries, individuals honor their needs, values, and limitations, fostering a deeper connection with themselves and cultivating a sense of inner peace.

Facilitating Spiritual Growth: Boundaries are a foundation for spiritual growth and transformation in yoga practice. As individuals deepen their yoga practice, they become more attuned to their inner wisdom and intuition. Setting boundaries allows them to discern what supports their spiritual journey and what detracts from it, enabling them to make choices aligned with their highest purpose and evolution.

Creating Sacred Space: Boundaries create a sacred space where individuals can explore and expand their consciousness. Whether establishing boundaries in physical yoga practice (asana), meditation, or daily life interactions, creating a safe and nurturing environment supports exploring more profound layers of awareness and facilitates spiritual awakening.

From a Reiki Perspective

> *"Reiki is a way of being. It's not just a practice, but a way of living that involves taking care of yourself and others in a balanced way."*
> (Rand, 2005)

Preserving Energetic Integrity: In Reiki, a Japanese energy healing technique, boundaries are closely tied to preserving energetic integrity. Practitioners learn to establish boundaries to protect their energy field (aura) from external influences and to maintain a clear channel for the flow of universal life force energy (ki or chi). Clear boundaries ensure that practitioners remain grounded, centered, and receptive to the healing energies of Reiki.

Respecting Client Autonomy: Reiki practitioners honor their clients' autonomy and free will by setting boundaries around the therapeutic relationship. This includes obtaining informed consent before offering Reiki treatment, respecting clients' physical and emotional boundaries during sessions, and maintaining confidentiality and professionalism. Clear boundaries create a safe and empowering space for clients to receive healing and support their journey of self-discovery.

Promoting Self-Care for Practitioners: Setting boundaries is essential for Reiki practitioners' well-being. Practicing self-care involves knowing when to say no to excessive demands on their time and energy, prioritizing their self-healing and spiritual practice, and establishing healthy boundaries in relationships with clients, colleagues, and others in their personal and professional lives.

Enhancing the Effectiveness of Reiki: Boundaries play a role in enhancing the effectiveness of Reiki practice. By maintaining clear boundaries, practitioners create a focused and intentional space for healing, free from distractions or interference. This allows the healing energy of Reiki to flow freely and facilitates deep relaxation, stress reduction, and holistic well-being for both the practitioner and the recipient.

Boundaries are essential for personal growth and well-being from both Yogic and Reiki perspectives. They help individuals maintain energetic balance, honor their own needs and values, facilitate spiritual growth and transformation, create sacred space for healing, preserve energetic integrity, respect client autonomy, promote self-care for practitioners, and enhance the effectiveness of Reiki practice. Individuals can navigate life's challenges with greater clarity, resilience, and compassion by cultivating healthy boundaries, leading to a more profound sense of harmony and fulfillment.

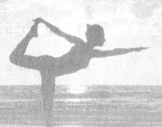

CHAPTER 3

The Eight Limbs of Yoga and the Principles of Reiki

The Eight Limbs of Yoga

The Eight Limbs of Yoga, as outlined in the Yoga Sutras of Patanjali, provide a comprehensive framework for achieving union (yoga) with oneself and the universe. Each limb guides ethical living, self-discipline, physical practice, and spiritual growth. Here's how each limb can inform the setting of boundaries.

> "The restraint of the modification of the mind-stuff is Yoga' (*Yoga Sutras* 1.2)."

The first two limbs, Yama and Niyama, are unique as they hold different offshoots. Yama and Niyama are the ethical foundations of yoga, providing guidelines for interacting with the world and oneself. Yama focuses on social conduct and the principles of ethical restraints, while Niyamas emphasizes personal observance. Together, they form the moral compass for a balanced and harmonious life.

1. The Yamas (Ethical Restraints)

Ahimsa (Non-violence): Setting boundaries rooted in non-violence involves refraining from harming oneself or others. This includes avoiding physical, verbal, or emotional aggression and cultivating compassion and empathy in interactions with oneself and others.

Satya (Truthfulness): Boundaries founded on truthfulness entail being honest and authentic in expressing one's needs, values, and limitations. This fosters transparency and trust in relationships, allowing for open communication and mutual understanding.

Asteya (Non-stealing): Setting boundaries with non-stealing means respecting others' time, energy, and resources while honoring one's boundaries. It involves establishing clear expectations and boundaries around personal space, belongings, and energy exchanges.

Brahmacharya (Moderation): Practicing moderation and self-restraint, particularly in sensory pleasures, encourages using energy wisely and avoiding excessive indulgence. Boundary setting means creating limits that prevent overextension and maintain personal energy.

Aparigraha (Non-possessiveness): Letting go of attachment and the desire to possess. It involves embracing generosity and simplicity and not holding on to physical or emotional clutter.

2. Niyamas (Observances)

Saucha (Purity): Boundaries rooted in purity involve creating a clean and sacred space within oneself and one's environment. This includes setting boundaries around self-care practices, maintaining a clutter-free physical space, and cultivating mental clarity and emotional balance.

Santosha (Contentment): Setting boundaries from a place of contentment involves accepting oneself and one's circumstances without constantly seeking external validation or approval. It entails establishing boundaries and prioritizing inner peace and fulfillment over external validation or approval.

Tapas (Self-Discipline): Boundaries informed by self-discipline involve honoring commitments to oneself and others, even when it requires saying no or setting limits. This entails setting boundaries around time management, energy expenditure, and personal goals to maintain focus and dedication.

Svadhyaya (Self-Study): plays a crucial role in boundary setting by encouraging deep reflection and self-awareness. Through the practice of Svadhyaya, we gain insight into our true selves, recognizing our needs, values, and limitations. This heightened self-awareness allows us to identify and establish boundaries that protect our well-being and align with our authentic selves. By regularly engaging in self-reflection, we can reassess and adjust our boundaries as needed, ensuring they continue to support our personal growth and maintain healthy relationships. We use sacred text and timeless spiritual law for guidance as we explore the depths of our life's journey.

Ishvara Pranidhana (Surrender to a Higher Power): helps set boundaries by encouraging trust and acceptance in the flow of life. This practice invites us to recognize our limitations and release the need to control everything, which can often lead to stress and overextension. By surrendering to a higher power, we cultivate humility and discernment, allowing us to establish boundaries that honor our well-being and the natural order of things. This surrender fosters a sense of peace and balance, enabling us to create and maintain boundaries that support our spiritual and emotional health.

3. Asanas (Physical Postures): While physical postures in yoga primarily focus on the physical body, they also indirectly support boundary-setting by promoting self-awareness, selfcare, and bodily autonomy. Engaging in yoga asanas can help individuals connect with their bodies, identify physical limitations, and cultivate a sense of empowerment in setting boundaries around physical comfort and safety.

4. Pranayama (Breath Control): Pranayama practices cultivate awareness of the breath and its connection to the mind and emotions. Setting boundaries informed by pranayama involves using breathwork to regulate stress responses, manage emotions, and create space for clarity and discernment in decision-making.

5. Pratyahara (Withdrawal of the Senses): Pratyahara invites individuals to turn inward and withdraw from external distractions to cultivate inner awareness and mindfulness. Setting boundaries through pratyahara involves creating space for introspection, reflection, and self-inquiry, allowing individuals to discern their needs and values and set boundaries aligned with their authentic selves.

6. Dharana (Concentration): Dharana practices develop the ability to focus the mind and concentrate on a single point of awareness. Setting boundaries through Dharana involves directing attention and energy toward clear intentions, priorities, and boundaries, fostering mental clarity, and resolving personal boundaries.

7. Dhyana (Meditation): Meditation deepens the state of inward awareness and connection with the present moment. Setting boundaries through meditation involves cultivating a sense of inner calm and serenity, which supports the ability to discern and maintain healthy boundaries amidst external pressures and distractions.

8. Samadhi (Bliss): Samadhi represents the state of transcendence and unity with the divine or universal consciousness. Setting boundaries from a place of samadhi involves recognizing the interconnectedness of all beings and setting boundaries that honor the inherent dignity and worth of oneself and others, fostering harmony and compassion in relationships.

Reiki Principles

The principles of Reiki, as articulated by its founder Mikao Usui, offer moral guidelines for living a balanced and harmonious life. Mikao Usui is quoted as saying, "Just for today, do not anger; do not worry; be grateful; be honest in your work; be compassionate to yourself and others." (Rand, 1991) These principles emphasize mindfulness, gratitude, integrity, and compassion. Here's how each principle can inform boundary-setting:

Just for today, do not anger: Setting boundaries from a place of non-anger involves approaching boundary-setting with calmness, compassion, and emotional intelligence. It entails refraining from reacting impulsively or aggressively and responding to boundary violations with clarity and assertiveness while maintaining respect for oneself and others.

Just for today, do not worry: Setting boundaries informed by non-worry involves releasing anxiety and fear surrounding boundary-setting and trusting in one's ability to prioritize self-care and well-being. It entails letting go of the need for external validation or approval and focusing on honoring one's needs and values in setting boundaries.

Just for today, be grateful: Setting boundaries from a place of gratitude involves appreciating oneself and others for their inherent worth and contributions. It entails recognizing the importance of self-respect and acknowledging the boundaries that support personal growth, well-being, and authenticity.

Just for today, be honest in your work: Setting boundaries with integrity involves aligning actions with values and commitments, even when it requires courage or discomfort. It entails honoring agreements, respecting others' boundaries, and communicating honestly and transparently in setting and upholding personal boundaries.

Just for today, be compassionate to yourself and others: Setting boundaries from a place of kindness involves approaching boundary-setting with empathy, compassion, and respect for oneself and others. It entails recognizing the interconnectedness of all beings and setting boundaries that promote mutual understanding, harmony, and well-being in relationships.

The five Reiki Principles emphasize the importance of self-compassion and mindfulness, essential in setting and maintaining healthy boundaries. Reiki promotes releasing negative energy and attachments, allowing for a freer, more open state of being. In terms of boundaries, it means not clinging to unhealthy relationships or situations.

In summary, both the Eight Limbs of Yoga and the principles of Reiki offer valuable frameworks for setting boundaries that promote personal growth, well-being, and harmonious relationships. By integrating the ethical principles and practices of Yoga and Reiki into boundary-setting, individuals can cultivate greater self-awareness, compassion, and authenticity in honoring their own needs and values while fostering mutual respect and understanding in relationships with others.

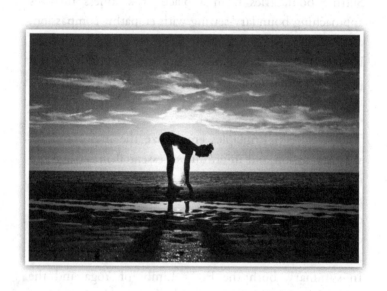

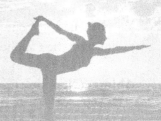

CHAPTER 4

Boundaries through Yamas (Ethical Restraints) and Reiki Principles

The Yamas, the first limb of the Eight Limbs of Yoga, serve as ethical restraints that encourage us to live in harmony with others and ourselves. These principles—Ahimsa (non-violence), Satya (truthfulness), Asteya (non-stealing), Brahmacharya (moderation), and Aparigraha (non-possessiveness)—provide a foundation for setting healthy boundaries. By embracing these ethical practices, we cultivate respect, integrity, and compassion in our interactions, which are essential for establishing and maintaining boundaries that honor our well-being and those around us.

The Yamas consist of ethical guidelines or restraining practices designed to guide interactions with the world. These principles promote harmonious living by encouraging non-violence, truthfulness, non-stealing, moderation, and non-possessiveness. By integrating these ethical practices with the principles of Reiki, individuals can create and maintain healthy boundaries that support personal growth and respectful relationships. Below, we explore how each

Yama can help set boundaries and provide practical scenarios to illustrate their application.

Ahimsa (Non-violence) and Reiki Compassion

Ahimsa: Ahimsa encourages non-violence and compassion towards oneself and others. It teaches individuals to refrain from physically, emotionally, or energetically harming others.

Reiki Compassion: Reiki principles emphasize compassion and loving-kindness as fundamental healing aspects. Practicing Reiki involves channeling universal life force energy with pure intention and unconditional love.

Integration: Understanding boundaries through Ahimsa and Reiki principles involves approaching boundary-setting with compassion and empathy. It entails recognizing the importance of honoring one's own needs and limits while respecting the autonomy and well-being of others.

Satya (Truthfulness) and Reiki Ethics

Satya: Satya encourages truthfulness and honesty in thoughts, words, and actions. It involves aligning with one's inner truth and expressing it authentically.

Reiki Ethics: Reiki practitioners adhere to ethical guidelines that promote integrity, transparency, and respect for the client's autonomy and confidentiality.

Integration: Understanding boundaries through Satya and Reiki ethics entails communicating boundaries honestly and clearly. It involves being truthful about one's needs, preferences, and limitations while upholding ethical standards of respect and integrity in interpersonal interactions.

Asteya (Non-stealing) and Reiki Trust

Asteya: Asteya encourages non-stealing and integrity in all aspects of life, including respecting others' possessions, time, and energy.

Reiki Trust: Reiki fosters trust in the healing process and the innate wisdom of the body-mind-spirit system. Practitioners trust in the natural flow of Reiki energy and the client's ability to receive and integrate it.

Integration: Understanding boundaries through Asteya and Reiki trust involves respecting personal boundaries and consent. It requires refraining from taking advantage of others' time, energy, or resources without permission while trusting in the mutual exchange of healing energy and respecting the client's autonomy in the Reiki healing process.

Brahmacharya (Moderation) and Reiki Harmony

Brahmacharya: Brahmacharya advocates for moderation, self-restraint, and balanced use of energy, particularly in the context of relationships and sensory indulgence.

Reiki Harmony: Reiki promotes energetic balance and harmony within oneself and with others. It encourages individuals to cultivate a harmonious relationship with themselves, others, and the universe.

Integration: Understanding boundaries through Brahmacharya and Reiki harmony involves maintaining balance and integrity in relationships. It requires discerning when to engage and when to withdraw, setting boundaries around personal space, time, and energy while fostering harmonious connections based on mutual respect and balance.

Aparigraha (Non-attachment) and Reiki Surrender

Aparigraha: Aparigraha encourages non-attachment and letting go of possessiveness or grasping tendencies. It teaches individuals to release attachment to outcomes and embrace impermanence.

Reiki Surrender: Reiki practice involves surrendering to the flow of universal life force energy and trusting in the innate healing intelligence of the body-mind-spirit complex.

Integration: Understanding boundaries through Aparigraha and Reiki surrender involves releasing attachment to control and allowing for organic growth and transformation. It entails setting boundaries with flexibility and openness, acknowledging that boundaries may evolve in response to changing circumstances and inner guidance.

Understanding boundaries through Yamas and Reiki principles invites individuals to cultivate a holistic approach to boundary-setting that integrates compassion, truthfulness, integrity, trust, balance, and surrender. It empowers individuals to establish boundaries that honor their authenticity, well-being, and interconnectedness with others and the universe.

An Example of How to Apply the Yamas and Reiki Principles to Set Boundaries

Scenario: Henry is a dedicated employee at a bustling restaurant known for its delicious cuisine and exceptional customer service. However, Henry often feels drained and overwhelmed by the demands of his job, struggling to maintain a healthy work-life balance. He recognizes that he needs to establish clearer boundaries to prioritize his well-being while still excelling in his career.

Ahimsa (Non-violence) and Reiki Compassion

Challenge: Henry often feels pressured to take extra shifts or cover for colleagues, fearing that saying no will disappoint his coworkers or harm his reputation.

Solution: Henry learns to prioritize self-care without guilt or self-judgment by practicing Ahimsa and Reiki compassion. He understands that setting boundaries is essential for his overall health and effectiveness while maintaining compassion for his coworkers' needs.

Satya (Truthfulness) and Reiki Ethics

Challenge: Henry needs to work on communicating his boundaries assertively, fearing that he will be perceived as uncooperative or unreliable.

Solution: Through Satya and Reiki ethics, Henry learns to communicate his needs and limitations honestly and respectfully. He understands that clear and transparent communication is crucial for maintaining healthy working relationships and mutual respect.

Asteya (Non-stealing) and Reiki Trust

Challenge: Henry often sacrifices his personal time and energy to meet the demands of his job, neglecting his own needs and well-being.

Solution: By practicing Asteya and Reiki's trust, Henry learns to value his time and energy as precious resources. He sets boundaries around his availability and commits to honoring his personal and professional commitments with integrity and balance.

Brahmacharya (Moderation) and Reiki Harmony

Challenge: Henry needs help finding a balance between his work responsibilities and personal life, often feeling overwhelmed and stressed.

Solution: Through Brahmacharya and Reiki harmony, Henry learns to prioritize self-care and create boundaries around his work schedule. He establishes dedicated time for rest, relaxation, and personal hobbies, fostering a sense of balance and harmony in his life.

Aparigraha (Non-attachment) and Reiki Surrender

Challenge: Henry becomes attached to outcomes and perfectionism, fearing failure or criticism if he doesn't meet expectations.

Solution: By practicing Aparigraha and Reiki surrender, Henry learns to release attachment to outcomes and embrace imperfection. He understands that setting boundaries is about doing his best while letting go of unrealistic expectations and allowing for growth and learning in his career.

Outcome: Through integrating Yamas and Reiki principles, Henry experiences a profound shift in his approach to boundary-setting and self-care in the food service industry. He learns to prioritize his well-being while still delivering exceptional service to customers and supporting his coworkers. Henry feels empowered to communicate his boundaries confidently, knowing that doing so is essential for his health, happiness, and professional success.

The unfortunate reality is that advocating for oneself in a toxic workplace can sometimes lead to negative consequences, such as being unfairly fired. This reflects a broader truth in boundary-setting: we cannot control other people's reactions, and trying to do so would be a form of violence against our integrity. However, living in fear of retribution does not align with our needs or values. In no way would forgoing his boundaries and continuing to suffer at his job be a better outcome for Henry. His work setting boundaries may also involve preparing himself emotionally and materially for potential fallout while releasing any sense of self-blame if such an outcome occurs. This process is about honoring his well-being and understanding that while he cannot control others' actions, he can control how he responds to them.

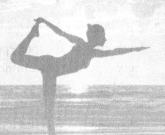

CHAPTER 5

Ahimsa (Non-Violence) and Reiki Precepts

Ahimsa, a concept rooted in Hindu, Buddhist, and Jain traditions, encapsulates the principle of non-violence towards all living beings. In energy healing practices like Reiki, this principle finds resonance in the Reiki Precepts, which guide practitioners in living a life of balance and harmony. In this chapter, we delve into the intersection of Ahimsa and the Reiki Precepts, mainly focusing on setting boundaries with compassion and non-harm.

Ahimsa (Non-Violence): Ahimsa, derived from Sanskrit, translates to 'non-violence' or 'non-harm.' It's not merely abstaining from physical violence but extends to one's thoughts, words, and actions. Ahimsa invites us to cultivate empathy, kindness, and compassion towards all beings, fostering harmony within ourselves and the world around us.

The Reiki Precepts: Reiki is guided by the five principles outlined in Chapter 3, known as the Reiki Precepts. These precepts serve as moral guidelines for Reiki practitioners, promoting spiritual growth and inner peace. While different versions of the precepts exist, they generally emphasize concepts like peacefulness, mindfulness, gratitude, integrity, and compassion.

Setting Boundaries with Compassion: Setting boundaries is crucial for maintaining healthy relationships and personal well-being. However, setting boundaries can sometimes be challenging, especially when it involves saying no or asserting oneself. By intertwining the principles of Ahimsa and the Reiki Precepts, we can approach boundary-setting with compassion and non-harm.

Non-Violence in Communication: When establishing boundaries, communication plays a pivotal role. Practicing Ahimsa in communication involves expressing oneself honestly and assertively while refraining from aggressive or hurtful language. By embodying the first precept of Reiki—abstaining from anger—we can communicate our boundaries with a calm and compassionate demeanor.

Cultivating Empathy: Empathy lies at the heart of Ahimsa and the Reiki Precepts. Before setting boundaries, it's essential to empathize with the perspectives and feelings of others involved. By embracing the fifth Reiki Precept—being kind to every living thing—we can approach boundary-setting with understanding and compassion, recognizing the humanity in ourselves and others.

Honoring Self-Care: Setting boundaries is an act of self-care, affirming our worth, and prioritizing our well-being. By aligning with the second and third Reiki

Precepts—refraining from worry and cultivating gratitude—we can approach boundary-setting from a self-awareness and appreciation for our needs.

Respecting Others' Boundaries: Just as we set boundaries for ourselves, it's essential to respect the boundaries of others. Practicing Ahimsa means honoring the autonomy and dignity of every individual, even when their boundaries may differ from ours. By embodying the fourth Reiki Precept—doing our work honestly—we can navigate relationships with integrity and respect.

In the intersection of Ahimsa and the Reiki Precepts lies a profound wisdom that guides us in setting boundaries with compassion and non-harm. By embracing these principles, we can create relationships built on empathy, respect, and understanding, fostering harmony within ourselves and the world around us. As we navigate the complexities of human interaction, may we always strive to embody the spirit of Ahimsa, nurturing a world where boundaries are set with love and kindness.

Setting Boundaries with Compassion and Non-harm Using the Principles of Ahimsa and the Reiki Precepts

Workplace Boundaries: Imagine you're in a work environment where your workload is consistently overwhelming, leading to stress and burnout. Instead of silently enduring the situation, you set boundaries by expressing your concerns to your supervisor. You approach the conversation with empathy, acknowledging the demands they face, but also assertively communicate your limitations and the need for a more manageable workload. By embodying the principles of Ahimsa and the Reiki Precepts, you advocate for yourself while maintaining respect and understanding for your supervisor's perspective.

Social Boundaries: Suppose you have a friend who often crosses boundaries by making insensitive comments or invading your personal space. Rather than ignoring their behavior or reacting angrily, you address the issue calmly and compassionately. You express how their actions impact you, emphasizing the importance of mutual respect in your friendship. By embodying the Reiki Precepts of kindness and honesty, you nurture the relationship while setting clear boundaries that uphold your well-being.

Family Boundaries: In a family setting, you may encounter situations where certain relatives overstep boundaries, whether it's offering unsolicited advice or prying into personal matters. Instead of resorting to confrontation or withdrawal, you practice Ahimsa by approaching the situation with understanding and empathy. You communicate your boundaries gently yet firmly, emphasizing your need for autonomy and privacy while reaffirming your love and respect for your family members.

Self-Care Boundaries: Consider a scenario where you constantly feel obligated to accommodate others' needs at the expense of your well-being. Recognizing the importance of self-care, you decide to set boundaries by prioritizing your needs and saying no when necessary. Whether declining extra work assignments or carving out time for self-care activities, you honor your boundaries with compassion and integrity, knowing that self-care is essential for your overall health and happiness.

Online Boundaries: Maintaining boundaries online is equally important in the digital age. Suppose you encounter online harassment or negativity on social media platforms. Instead of engaging in heated arguments or retaliating with hostility, you choose to disengage from toxic interactions and block or report abusive users. By embodying the Reiki Precepts of non-anger and kindness, you protect your mental well-being while promoting a culture of respect and positivity in online communities.

These examples illustrate how Ahimsa and the Reiki Precepts principles can guide us in setting boundaries with compassion and non-harm in various aspects of life. By prioritizing empathy, honesty, and self-respect, we can cultivate healthier relationships, maintain our well-being, and contribute to a more harmonious world.

Ahimsa and the Reiki Precepts principles can help you navigate setting boundaries with compassion and non-harm, fostering healthier relationships and greater well-being.

Self-Reflection and Awareness: Take time to reflect on your own needs, values, and boundaries. Consider areas where you feel overextended or where boundaries have been crossed. Cultivate self-awareness by tuning into your emotions, physical sensations, and inner guidance. Notice how specific interactions or situations affect your well-being.

Clarify Your Boundaries: Identify specific areas where you need to set boundaries, whether in relationships, work, social activities, or personal time. Clearly define what behaviors or actions are acceptable and unacceptable to you. Be specific about your boundaries and the consequences of crossing them.

Communicate with Compassion: Approach boundary-setting conversations with empathy and compassion for yourself and others involved. Use "I" statements to express your feelings and needs without blaming or accusing others. For example, "I feel overwhelmed when..." or "I need to prioritize my self-care by..." Practice active listening, allowing others to express their perspectives without judgment. Validate their feelings while staying firm in asserting your boundaries.

Enforce Boundaries with Firmness and Respect: Be firm and consistent in upholding your boundaries, even if it feels uncomfortable or met with resistance. Use assertive communication techniques to stand your ground while maintaining respect for others. Avoid aggression, passive-aggressiveness, or manipulation. Set consequences for boundary violations and follow through with them when necessary. This reinforces the importance of respecting boundaries and establishes accountability.

Practice Self-Compassion and Self-Care: Be gentle with yourself as you navigate the process of setting boundaries. It's okay to feel uncomfortable or uncertain, mainly if you're not accustomed to prioritizing your needs. Practice self-care regularly to nurture your physical, emotional, and spiritual well-being. Make time for activities that replenish your energy and bring you joy. Remember that setting boundaries is an act of self-love and self-respect. Honor your boundaries as a way of honoring yourself.

Review and Adjust as Needed: Review your boundaries periodically to ensure they align with your needs and values. Life circumstances may change, requiring adjustments to your boundaries. Be open to feedback from trusted friends, family members, or mentors who can offer perspective and support. Celebrate your progress and growth in honoring your boundaries, recognizing that it's a journey of self-discovery and empowerment.

An Example of Setting Boundaries with Compassion and Non-Harm in a Workplace

Setting boundaries in the workplace is crucial for maintaining a healthy work-life balance and ensuring personal well-being. However, doing so with compassion and non-harm can be challenging, especially when communicating with supervisors or colleagues. By integrating the principles of yoga and Reiki, individuals can navigate these conversations with clarity, empathy, and respect. The following scenario illustrates how one might approach setting boundaries compassionately and non-harmfully.

Scenario: Christina has been feeling overwhelmed with her workload for several weeks. Despite her best efforts, she finds it challenging to keep up with her tasks, which is affecting her mental and physical health. She decides to approach her supervisor, Mark, to discuss her concerns and set some boundaries to manage her workload better. Drawing on the principles of Ahimsa (non-violence) and Satya (truthfulness) from the Yamas, Christina prepares to communicate her needs honestly and respectfully, ensuring that her approach is constructive and compassionate.

Christina: Hi, Mark. Do you have a moment to chat?

Mark: Sure, Christina. What's on your mind?

Christina: I wanted to talk to you about my workload. I've been feeling overwhelmed with the number of projects on my plate.

Mark: I see. I know we've had a lot going on recently. What specifically has been causing you to feel overwhelmed?

Christina: I've been juggling multiple deadlines simultaneously, and keeping up has been challenging. I've been working late hours and even on weekends to meet all the demands, but I'm starting to feel burned out.

Mark: I appreciate you bringing this to my attention, Christina. Your well-being is important to me. Is there anything specific that's contributing to the workload pressure? Are there tasks that could be delegated or deadlines that could be adjusted?

Christina: Part of it is the volume of tasks, but some deadlines feel unrealistic given the scope of the projects. It's challenging to maintain a healthy work-life balance.

Mark: I understand. I'll look closer at the deadlines and see if there's room for adjustments. In the meantime, it's okay to prioritize your well-being. Your health and happiness are essential; I don't want you to feel overwhelmed or burnt out.

Christina: Thank you, Mark. I appreciate your understanding. I propose setting more realistic deadlines and redistributing some of the workload. It would allow me to maintain a better balance and perform at my best.

Mark: That sounds like a reasonable approach. Let's work together to develop a plan supporting your well-being while ensuring our projects are completed effectively. I value your contributions to the team, Christina, and I want to make sure you feel supported in your role.

Christina: Thank you, Mark. I feel relieved knowing that we can address this together. I'm committed to doing my best work, and with these adjustments, I can contribute even more effectively to the team.

Mark: Absolutely, Christina. We're in this together, and I'm here to support you every step of the way. Let's schedule a follow-up meeting to discuss the proposed changes and how to implement them.

Christina: Sounds good. Thanks again, Mark.

Outcome: Christina approaches her supervisor, Mark, with honesty and vulnerability, expressing her feelings of overwhelm and burnout. Mark responds with empathy and understanding, validating Christina's concerns and offering support. Together, they collaborate on finding solutions that prioritize Christina's well-being while also addressing the demands of the workload. This conversation demonstrates how setting boundaries with compassion and non-harm can foster open communication, mutual respect, and positive outcomes in a professional setting.

An Example of Setting Boundaries Using Ahimsa and the Reiki Precepts in a Friendship

Maintaining healthy boundaries in friendships is essential for fostering mutual respect and understanding. When a friend's behavior causes emotional distress, addressing the issue with compassion and non-harm can help preserve the relationship while protecting one's well-being. Individuals can navigate these sensitive conversations with care and empathy by applying the principle of Ahimsa (non-violence) from yoga and the Reiki Precepts. The following scenario demonstrates how one might constructively set boundaries in a friendship to address hurtful behavior.

Scenario: Alex has been feeling increasingly hurt by Jamie's constant criticism, which has started to take a toll on their self-esteem and the overall quality of their friendship. To address this, Alex has an open and honest conversation with Jamie. Guided by Ahimsa (non-violence) and the Reiki Precepts, Alex aims to communicate their feelings without causing harm, fostering a space for understanding and positive change.

Alex: Hey Jamie, can we talk for a moment?

Jamie: Sure, what's up?

Alex: I wanted to chat about something on my mind lately. I've noticed that sometimes you make comments that feel critical or judgmental when we're hanging out, and it's been bothering me.

Jamie: Oh, I didn't realize. I'm sorry if I've said anything that hurt you. Can you give me some examples?

Alex: Well, for instance, the other day, when we talked about my job, you commented on how I could be doing more to advance my career. It made me feel like you were criticizing my choices, even though I'm happy with where I am.

Jamie: I see. I didn't mean to come across that way. I was just trying to offer some advice, but I can see how it sounded judgmental.

Alex: I appreciate that you were trying to help, but sometimes I just need you to listen and support me without offering advice or criticism. I know you care about me, and I value your input, but it's vital for me to feel respected and accepted for who I am.

Jamie: I understand, Alex. I'll make a conscious effort to be more mindful of how I communicate with you and offer support in a way that feels helpful. I don't want to make you feel uncomfortable or judged in any way.

Alex: Thank you, Jamie. I appreciate that. Our friendship means a lot to me, and I want us to be open and honest without fear of judgment.

Jamie: Absolutely, Alex. I value our friendship, too, and I'm committed to respecting your boundaries and supporting you in the way you need. Let's keep the lines of communication open and check in with each other regularly.

Alex: Sounds good. Thanks for being understanding, Jamie.

Outcome: When Alex initiates a dialogue with Jamie about their feelings of hurt and discomfort regarding Jamie's critical comments, Jamie responds with empathy and apologizes for any unintentional harm caused. They engage in a constructive conversation about setting boundaries for communication within their friendship, with Alex expressing the need for support and acceptance without judgment. Jamie acknowledges Alex's boundaries and commits to respecting them moving forward. This conversation demonstrates how setting personal boundaries with compassion and non-harm can strengthen friendships and foster mutual understanding and respect.

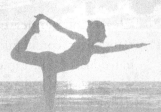

CHAPTER 6

Satya (Truthfulness) and Reiki Ethics

Satya, or truthfulness, is one of the Yamas (ethical restraints) in the Eight Limbs of Yoga, while authentic communication is an essential aspect of Reiki ethics. Let's explore how Satya and Reiki ethics intersect in honoring personal truth and communicating boundaries authentically.

Satya (Truthfulness): Satya involves being honest and authentic in thoughts, words, and actions. It goes beyond simply refraining from lying and encompasses speaking the truth with kindness and integrity. Satya encourages individuals to acknowledge and express their genuine needs, feelings, and values when setting boundaries. Here's how Satya can inform boundary-setting:

Self-Reflection: Satya begins with self-awareness and self-honesty. Before setting boundaries, individuals need to reflect on their needs, limitations, and values. This introspection helps them identify where boundaries are needed and what boundaries align with their authentic selves.

Clear Communication: Satya emphasizes clear and transparent communication. When setting boundaries, individuals should express themselves honestly and directly, without fear of judgment or rejection. This means clearly stating their needs, expectations, and limits while respecting the needs and boundaries of others.

Authenticity: Satya encourages authenticity in relationships. Setting boundaries authentically means being true to oneself and honoring one's truth, even if it may be uncomfortable or unpopular. Authentic boundary-setting fosters genuine connections and promotes mutual respect and understanding.

Respect for Others: Satya also involves respecting others' truths. When communicating boundaries, individuals should do so with empathy and compassion, recognizing that others may have different perspectives and needs. Honoring the truth of others while asserting one's boundaries promotes healthy and harmonious relationships.

Reiki Ethics: Reiki ethics encompass a set of moral principles and guidelines that Reiki practitioners adhere to, emphasizing integrity, respect, and compassion in all aspects of Reiki healing. Regarding boundary-setting, Reiki ethics provide a framework for honoring personal truth and communicating boundaries authentically. Here's how Reiki ethics intersect with Satya in boundary-setting.

Integrity: Reiki ethics emphasize the importance of integrity and honesty in all interactions. Reiki practitioners should do so with integrity when setting boundaries and aligning their actions with true intentions and values. This means being genuine and transparent in expressing boundaries and avoiding manipulation or deceit.

Respect for Autonomy: Reiki ethics prioritize respecting clients' autonomy and free will. When communicating boundaries in a Reiki session, practitioners should do so in a way that honors the client's right to make their own choices and decisions. This may involve explaining the purpose and significance of certain boundaries and seeking the client's consent and cooperation.

Compassionate Communication: Reiki ethics encourage compassionate and empathetic communication. When setting boundaries, practitioners should communicate with kindness and sensitivity, considering the feelings and needs of the client. This helps build trust and rapport and fosters a supportive and healing environment.

Self-Care: Reiki ethics highlight the importance of self-care for practitioners. Setting boundaries is an act of self-care, allowing practitioners to maintain their own well-being and energy balance. Practitioners should honor their truth and boundaries, even limiting the number of clients they see or the type of sessions they offer.

These aspects of Satya and Reiki ethics have translated into effective boundary-setting for clients across various industries. These principles of truthfulness, energy protection, and compassionate self-awareness have proven valuable beyond the realm of Reiki, offering guidance for professionals in maintaining integrity and balance in diverse personal and professional contexts.

Honoring Personal Truth and Communicating Boundaries Authentically

When combining Satya from yoga philosophy with Reiki ethics, individuals can effectively honor their truth and communicate boundaries authentically in Reiki practice and beyond. This involves:

Self-awareness and introspection: Reflecting on one's needs, values, and boundaries.

Clear and transparent communication: Expressing boundaries honestly and directly while respecting the autonomy and feelings of others.

Acting with integrity and compassion: Setting boundaries with integrity, empathy, and kindness in alignment with one's true intentions and values.

Prioritizing self-care: Honoring personal boundaries and self-care needs, even in the context of healing and helping others.

By integrating the principles of Satya and Reiki ethics into boundary-setting, individuals can cultivate deeper self-awareness, strengthen relationships, and promote overall well-being and harmony.

An Example of Setting Boundaries Using Satya and Reiki Ethics in a Family Dynamic

Scenario: Sophia is a mother who struggles with maintaining boundaries with her teenage daughter, Emily. Emily frequently disregards curfews and spends excessive time on her phone, causing tension and conflict in their relationship. Sophia realizes the importance of setting boundaries to foster mutual respect and understanding while promoting Emily's well-being.

Self-awareness and Authenticity: Sophia reflects on her feelings of frustration and exhaustion resulting from the lack of boundaries with Emily. During her reflection, Sophia realizes she feels a combination of disrespect and fear. Sophia fears she doesn't know Emily as well as she once did because this stage of life has shifted their dynamic, and Sophia is worried about Emily's choices while she is out past curfew. Sophia feels disrespected because she believes Emily willfully disobeys her curfew. She acknowledges her role in enabling Emily's behavior by avoiding difficult conversations and setting clear expectations.

Clear and Compassionate Communication: Sophia decides to have an open and honest conversation with Emily about the importance of boundaries and mutual respect in their relationship. She expresses her concerns calmly and compassionately without blaming or criticizing Emily.

Respect for Autonomy: Sophia acknowledges Emily's autonomy and individuality while emphasizing the need for mutual respect and cooperation within the family.

She invites Emily to share her perspective and feelings, encouraging open dialogue and active listening.

Integrity and Self-Care: By asserting her boundaries with integrity and self-care, Sophia prioritizes her well-being and sets a positive example for Emily. She communicates her expectations regarding curfew and screen time, explaining the reasons behind these boundaries and the consequences for violating them.

Gratitude and Support: Sophia expresses her gratitude to Emily for her willingness to engage in the conversation and work together to establish healthy boundaries. She reassures Emily of her love and support while reinforcing the importance of mutual respect and accountability in their relationship.

Outcome: Through honest and compassionate communication grounded in Satya and Reiki ethics, Sophia and Emily can establish clear boundaries that promote harmony and understanding within their family. By honoring each other's truths and needs, they deepen their connection and strengthen their bond, fostering a supportive and nurturing environment for growth and well-being.

An Example of Setting Boundaries Using Satya and Reiki Ethics in a Professional Scenario

Scenario: Leanne is a social worker who is deeply committed to supporting her clients but often neglects her self-care. She realizes the importance of setting boundaries to prioritize her well-being and prevent burnout.

Self-awareness and Authenticity: Leanne acknowledges that she has overextended herself by taking on too many clients and neglecting her needs. She recognizes that this pattern is unsustainable and detrimental to her overall well-being.

Clear and Compassionate Communication: Leanne communicates her boundaries with her clients honestly and directly. She emails her clients explaining that she will be reducing her caseload and scheduling fewer appointments to prioritize her self-care and ensure the quality of her services.

Respect for Autonomy: Leanne emphasizes to her clients that she values their well-being and wants to provide the best possible support. She assures them that she will continue to honor existing appointments but may need to adjust future appointments to maintain her energy balance.

Integrity and Self-Care: By asserting her boundaries with integrity and self-care, Leanne prioritizes her well-being and sets a positive example for her clients. She recognizes that taking care of herself is essential to continue providing practical support and advocacy for her clients.

Gratitude and Support: Leanne appreciates her clients for their understanding and support. She reassures them that she remains committed to their well-being and will continue to provide her services with the same care and dedication, albeit with revised scheduling.

Outcome: Through honest and compassionate communication grounded in Satya and Reiki's ethical principles, Leanne can establish clear boundaries, prioritizing self-care while maintaining positive client relationships. By honoring her truth and needs, she creates a sustainable and fulfilling practice that promotes her overall well-being and supports her ability to continue serving others effectively in social work.

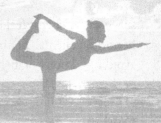

CHAPTER 7

Asteya (Non-stealing) and Reiki Ethics

Respecting Boundaries and Fostering Trust in Relationships

Asteya, the principle of non-stealing from the Yamas in yoga philosophy, emphasizes respecting the possessions, time, energy, and boundaries of others. When applied to Reiki ethics, it fosters trust and nurtures healthy relationships. Here's how Asteya and Reiki ethics intersect in respecting boundaries and fostering trust.

Respecting Personal Boundaries

Asteya: Asteya teaches us to avoid taking advantage of others' boundaries, possessions, or energy without consent. It involves respecting physical, emotional, and energetic boundaries and refraining from intruding upon them.

Reiki Ethics: Reiki ethics emphasize the importance of respecting the autonomy and well-being of clients. Practitioners are encouraged to create a safe, supportive space where clients feel respected and valued. This includes honoring clients' boundaries during Reiki sessions and avoiding actions or behaviors that may cause discomfort or distress.

Cultivating Trust

Asteya: By practicing Asteya, individuals demonstrate integrity and respect for others, which fosters trust and strengthens relationships. When people feel their boundaries are respected, they are more likely to trust and feel safe around others.

Reiki Ethics: Trust is fundamental in the Reiki relationship between practitioner and client. Practitioners must uphold ethical standards to build and maintain trust. This involves respecting clients' confidentiality, providing accurate information about Reiki practices, and ensuring a professional and supportive environment during sessions.

Communicating Boundaries

Asteya: Asteya encourages clear communication of boundaries to prevent misunderstandings or violations. Individuals are encouraged to assert their boundaries confidently and respectfully, allowing others to understand and honor them.

Reiki Ethics: Practitioners are encouraged to establish clear boundaries with clients regarding the nature and scope of Reiki sessions. This includes communicating any limitations or restrictions, obtaining informed consent before initiating touch or energy work, and addressing clients' concerns or questions about the process.

Promoting Reciprocity and Balance

Asteya: Asteya also involves giving back and contributing positively to others' well-being. It encourages a mindset of abundance rather than scarcity, where individuals recognize that there is enough for everyone and seek to support and uplift others.

Reiki Ethics: Reiki practitioners embody giving and receiving principles by maintaining a balanced energy exchange with clients. While practitioners offer healing energy during sessions, they also receive benefits such as personal growth, fulfillment, and gratitude from the healing process.

Upholding Ethical Standards

Asteya: Asteya guides individuals to adhere to ethical standards in their interactions with others, promoting fairness, honesty, and integrity in all dealings.

Reiki Ethics: Reiki ethics provide a framework for practitioners to uphold ethical standards in their practice, ensuring clients' well-being and best interests are prioritized. Practitioners are expected to conduct themselves with honesty, integrity, and professionalism.

By integrating the principles of Asteya and Reiki ethics, individuals can foster trust, respect boundaries, and nurture healthy, supportive relationships built on integrity, compassion, and mutual understanding. This enhances the effectiveness of Reiki sessions and promotes overall well-being and harmony in all interactions.

Examples of Professional and Personal Boundary Setting Incorporating the Principles of Asteya and Ethical Behavior

Scenario: Mark is a project manager leading a team on a tight deadline. He notices that one team member, David, consistently stays late to complete his work, often at the expense of his personal time and well-being.

Respecting Personal Boundaries: Mark recognizes that David's behavior may indicate a lack of work-life balance and respect for his boundaries. Mark refrains from expecting or encouraging David to work beyond reasonable hours and respects his right to prioritize his well-being.

Cultivating Trust: Mark fosters trust within the team by demonstrating integrity and respect for individual boundaries. By not pressuring David to overwork, Mark shows that he values the well-being of his team members and prioritizes their health and happiness over project deadlines.

Scenario: Jake and Ben are roommates sharing an apartment. Ben frequently borrows Jake's belongings without asking and sometimes needs to remember to return them promptly, causing Jake frustration.

Respecting Personal Boundaries: Jake acknowledges that Ben's behavior violates his boundaries and demonstrates a lack of respect for his possessions. Jake communicates his concerns to Ben, explaining the importance of asking for permission before borrowing items and returning them promptly.

Cultivating Trust: By addressing the issue with honesty and openness, Jake fosters trust and mutual respect in their roommate relationship. Ben recognizes the impact of his actions on Jake and commits to respecting his boundaries and possessions in the future, strengthening their trust and communication as roommates.

Outcome: In both examples, the individuals demonstrate Asteya by respecting personal boundaries and refraining from taking advantage of others. They nurture positive and harmonious relationships in both professional and personal contexts by upholding ethical behavior and promoting mutual respect, trust, and understanding.

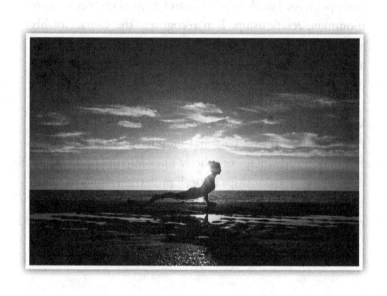

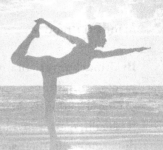

CHAPTER 8

Brahmacharya (Moderation) and Reiki Self-Care Guided Boundaries

Brahmacharya, often translated as moderation or celibacy, is one of the Yamas in yoga philosophy. It encourages individuals to cultivate self-control and balance in all aspects of life, including physical, emotional, and mental. When applied in conjunction with Reiki self-care, Brahmacharya can guide individuals in maintaining a balanced and harmonious energy flow within themselves. Here's how Brahmacharya and Reiki self-care intersect.

Brahmacharya: Brahmacharya encourages individuals to conserve and channel their energy wisely, avoiding excessive indulgence or depletion. It emphasizes moderation in all activities, including diet, sleep, work, and leisure.

Reiki Self-Care: Reiki self-care involves practicing techniques to balance and harmonize one's energy system. By incorporating Reiki principles and techniques into their daily routine, individuals can promote a balanced energy flow throughout their body, mind, and spirit.

Mindful Practice

Brahmacharya: Brahmacharya invites individuals to practice mindfulness and awareness in their daily activities, paying attention to their thoughts, emotions, and behaviors. It encourages individuals to cultivate self-control and discernment in their actions.

Reiki Self-Care: Reiki self-care involves practicing mindfulness and presence while performing Reiki techniques on oneself. By being fully present in the moment and attuned to their energy, individuals can deepen their self-awareness and facilitate healing and balance within themselves.

Setting Boundaries

Brahmacharya: Brahmacharya encourages individuals to set boundaries in their interactions and relationships, ensuring that others' demands or expectations do not deplete their energy. It involves saying no when necessary and prioritizing one's well-being.

Reiki Self-Care: Reiki self-care includes setting boundaries to protect one's energy and maintain balance. This may involve establishing a regular self-care practice, scheduling time for Reiki sessions, and prioritizing self-care activities that nurture and replenish one's energy.

Honoring the Body

Brahmacharya: Brahmacharya emphasizes the importance of honoring the body as a temple and treating it with respect and reverence. It involves adopting healthy lifestyle habits and avoiding harmful behaviors that deplete or disturb the body's natural balance.

Reiki Self-Care: Reiki self-care encourages individuals to honor their body's needs and listen to its signals. By practicing self-reiki and other self-care techniques, individuals can support their body's natural healing processes and maintain optimal health and vitality.

Cultivating Inner Peace

Brahmacharya: Brahmacharya leads to inner peace and contentment by fostering balance and moderation in all aspects of life. It allows individuals to transcend cravings and attachments, leading to inner harmony and tranquility.

Reiki Self-Care: Reiki self-care promotes inner peace and well-being by facilitating relaxation, stress reduction, and emotional healing. By regularly practicing Reiki, individuals can experience greater calmness, clarity, and serenity in their daily lives.

By integrating the principles of Brahmacharya with Reiki self-care, individuals can cultivate balance, harmony, and well-being on physical, emotional, and spiritual levels. This holistic approach to self-care empowers individuals to honor their body, mind, and spirit and live a life of moderation, mindfulness, and inner peace.

Examples of Brahmacharya and Reiki Self-Care in a Family and Personal Context

Scenario: The Johnson family consists of parents Alan and Sarah and their two children, Amy and Jack. They lead busy lives with work, school, and extracurricular activities but recognize the importance of maintaining balance and harmony within their family.

Family Time Moderation: The Johnson family practices moderation in their family time, ensuring a healthy balance of quality time together and individual pursuits. They schedule regular family activities such as game nights, outdoor outings, or shared meals but also respect each other's need for personal space and downtime.

Setting Boundaries: Each family member communicates their needs and boundaries openly and respectfully. For example, if one family member needs quiet time to recharge, they communicate this to the rest of the family, who then honor that boundary by giving them space and privacy.

Self-Care Practices: The Johnson family incorporates self-care practices into their daily routine to promote balance and well-being. They spend time together practicing breathwork, guided meditation, or relaxation techniques, fostering a sense of connection and mutual support.

Supporting Each Other: Family members support each other in their self-care practices and encourage each other to prioritize their well-being. For instance, if one family member is feeling stressed or overwhelmed, the rest of the family may offer encouragement, acts of kindness, or assistance with tasks to alleviate their burden.

Scenario: Brianna is a busy professional balancing her career, personal life, and self-care practices. She recognizes the importance of moderation and self-care to maintain balance and well-being.

Setting Boundaries: Brianna sets boundaries around her work hours, personal time, and social commitments to prevent burnout and maintain balance. She communicates her boundaries clearly to her colleagues, friends, and family, asserting her need for rest, relaxation, and self-care.

Moderating Activities: Brianna practices moderation in her daily activities by avoiding overcommitting herself and prioritizing activities that nourish her body, mind, and spirit. She schedules regular breaks throughout the day to rest, recharge, and engage in self-care practices such as meditation, journaling, or spending time in nature.

Reiki Self-Care Practices: Brianna incorporates Reiki self-care practices into her daily routine to promote relaxation, stress reduction, and emotional healing. She practices self-Reiki before bed to promote restful sleep and release any tension or stress accumulated throughout the day.

Nurturing Relationships: Brianna nurtures her relationships with loved ones, setting aside dedicated time for meaningful connections and quality time together. She communicates openly with her loved ones about self-care needs and encourages them to prioritize their well-being.

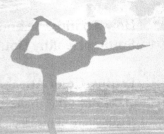

CHAPTER 9

Harnessing Aparigraha (Non-Attachment) and Reiki for Balance

Aparigraha, one of the five Yamas in the eight limbs of yoga, translates to non-possessiveness, non-greed, or non-attachment. This principle encourages us to relinquish our attachments to material possessions, people, and outcomes. It teaches us to live with what is necessary and to avoid the excesses that can clutter our lives and minds.

In Reiki, a practice focused on energy healing, a similar principle is applied to energy and emotional attachment. Reiki encourages practitioners to release negative energy and attachments that do not serve their highest good. By doing so, individuals can maintain a balanced and harmonious energy flow, essential for physical, emotional, and spiritual well-being.

How Aparigraha and Reiki Aid in Setting Healthy Boundaries

Letting Go of Attachment: Aparigraha teaches us to let go of our attachment to people, outcomes, and material possessions. This detachment allows us to set boundaries without guilt or fear of loss. We learn to understand that our worth is not tied to our possessions or the approval of others.

Energy Conservation: Reiki emphasizes the importance of maintaining a balanced energy flow. By letting go of attachments and negative energy, we conserve our energy for what truly matters. This energy conservation helps us establish boundaries that protect our well-being and prevent burnout.

Clarity and Focus: Both Aparigraha and Reiki practices promote mental clarity. By clearing out unnecessary attachments and energy blockages, we gain a clearer perspective on our needs and limits. This clarity is crucial in identifying and communicating our boundaries effectively.

Emotional Freedom: Releasing attachments and practicing non-possessiveness leads to emotional freedom. We become less reactive and more centered, which allows us to enforce boundaries calmly and assertively. This emotional stability is vital for maintaining healthy relationships and self-respect.

An Example of How to Apply Aparigraha and Reiki Principles in a Workplace

Scenario: John works in a high-pressure food service environment where he is constantly asked to take on extra shifts and responsibilities. Over time, this has led to burnout and a lack of personal time. He finds it hard to say no because he fears disappointing his colleagues and superiors.

Recognizing Attachment: John starts by acknowledging his attachment to the approval of others and the fear of being seen as inadequate. Through self-reflection, he understands that this attachment drains his energy and well-being.

Reiki Self-Healing: John begins practicing self-healing techniques to release the negative energy associated with his fear and attachment. He uses Reiki and meditation to balance his energy and promote emotional healing.

Setting Boundaries: With a clearer mind and balanced energy, John identifies his limits and the need for personal time. He communicates his boundaries to his manager, explaining that he can no longer take extra shifts without compromising his health.

Non-Possessiveness: Embracing Aparigraha, John lets go of the need for constant approval. He understands that his worth depends not on how much he can take on but on how well he cares for himself.

Consistent Practice: John continues to practice Reiki and Aparigraha regularly, reinforcing his boundaries and maintaining his energy balance. He notices an improvement in his well-being and a healthier work-life balance.

Aparigraha and Reiki offer powerful tools for setting healthy boundaries. By letting go of attachments and maintaining balanced energy, we can establish and uphold boundaries that protect our well-being and promote harmonious relationships. These practices encourage us to live with intention and clarity, making boundary-setting a natural and essential part of our lives.

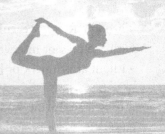

CHAPTER 10

Boundaries through Niyamas (Observances) and Reiki Practice

Setting boundaries with oneself is a profound journey of self-discovery and self-care, deeply rooted in the principles of Niyamas from yoga philosophy and Reiki practice. Niyamas, the second limb of yoga outlined by Patanjali in the Yoga Sutras, encompass personal observances guiding us towards inner harmony and spiritual growth. Reiki emphasizes the flow of universal life force energy for healing and balance. Integrating these principles offers a holistic approach to establishing boundaries that honor our true selves and promote well-being on all levels.

Saucha (Cleanliness and Purity): Setting boundaries with oneself begins with cultivating cleanliness and purity in our thoughts, emotions, and actions. In Reiki practice, we cleanse our energy channels and release stagnant energy to maintain purity and clarity in our energetic field.

Santosha (Contentment): Embracing contentment allows us to accept ourselves and recognize our inherent worthiness.

Through Reiki, we cultivate contentment by connecting with the present moment and accepting things as they are, without attachment or judgment.

Tapas (Discipline and Self-control): Tapas guides us to cultivate discipline and self-control to align with our values and intentions. In Reiki practice, we exercise discipline by committing to regular self-treatment and maintaining energetic boundaries to uphold our well-being.

Svadhyaya (Self-study and Self-reflection): Svadhyaya encourages self-awareness and introspection to understand our thoughts, emotions, and patterns. Through Reiki, we engage in self-reflection to uncover areas where boundaries may be needed, allowing us to honor our needs and values authentically.

Ishvara Pranidhana (Surrender to the Divine): Surrendering to the divine reminds us to trust in a higher power and relinquish control over outcomes. In Reiki practice, we surrender to the universal life force energy, allowing it to flow through us for healing and balance, trusting in its wisdom and guidance.

By integrating the principles of Niyamas and Reiki practice, we embark on self-discovery and empowerment, cultivating a deeper understanding of ourselves and our boundaries. We honor our true essence through mindfulness, self-reflection, and energetic alignment, creating space for growth, healing, and transformation. Setting boundaries with oneself becomes an act of self-love and self-respect, allowing us to live authentically and thrive in all aspects of our lives.

An Example of How to Set Boundaries with Oneself Using Niyamas and Reiki Practice

Scenario: Avery integrates the principles of Niyamas and Reiki practice into their step-by-step approach to setting boundaries with themself.

Saucha (Cleanliness and Purity): Avery begins their day with a Reiki self-treatment, cleansing their energy field and release any negativity accumulated from the previous day. They create a serene and clutter-free space in their home where they can engage in self-reflection and journaling, free from distractions. Avery reflects on recent interactions and notices patterns of overcommitting to others' needs at the expense of their well-being. In the spirit of ahimsa, Avery releases any resentment, anger, or frustration toward themselves or others. Avery recognizes the need for boundaries to maintain purity and clarity in their actions.

Santosha (Contentment): Avery practices gratitude meditation, focusing on the blessings in their life and cultivating a sense of contentment with who they are and where they are on their journey. They remind themselves that setting boundaries is an act of self-care and self-love, affirming their inherent worthiness and deservingness of respect.

Tapas (Discipline and Self-control): Avery establishes a daily routine that includes time for exercise, meditation, and Reiki practice, prioritizing their well-being and honoring their need for self-care. They commit to saying "no" to additional commitments or requests that do not align with their values or priorities, exercising discipline and self-control to maintain their boundaries.

Svadhyaya (Self-study and Self-reflection): Avery engages in journaling and mindfulness practices to gain insight into their thoughts, emotions, and behaviors, identifying areas where boundaries may be needed. They explore Reiki principles and teachings, seeking guidance on setting boundaries with compassion and self-awareness and uncovering any underlying beliefs or patterns that may hinder their ability to establish boundaries effectively.

Ishvara Pranidhana (Surrender to the Divine): Avery practices surrendering to the flow of universal life force energy, trusting in the wisdom of the divine to guide them in setting and maintaining healthy boundaries. They visualize themselves surrounded by a cocoon of healing light, surrendering fears or doubts about setting boundaries and trusting in self-discovery and growth.

Through this integrated approach, Avery empowers themself to set boundaries with compassion, self-awareness, and trust, fostering inner peace and well-being on their journey of self-discovery and personal growth.

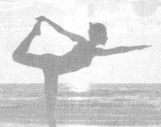

CHAPTER 11

Boundaries with Saucha (Purity) and Reiki Self-Cleansing

Let's delve deeper into the concepts of Saucha (Purity) and Reiki self-cleansing to provide a more comprehensive understanding of how they contribute to clearing mental clutter and prioritizing self-care boundaries.

Saucha (Purity): In yoga philosophy, Saucha, one of the Niyamas (personal observances), emphasizes purity and cleanliness in thoughts, emotions, and actions. It encourages individuals to cultivate clarity, simplicity, and integrity, promoting inner harmony and spiritual growth.

Mental Clarity: Saucha invites individuals to declutter their minds from negative thoughts, worries, and distractions that inhibit mental clarity and peace. By releasing mental clutter, one can experience more significant focus, presence, and well-being.

Emotional Balance: Saucha encourages individuals to purify their emotions by letting go of resentment, anger, and attachment. One can navigate life's challenges by fostering emotional balance with greater resilience, compassion, and serenity.

Physical Cleanliness: Saucha extends to physical cleanliness by promoting hygiene, organization, and orderliness in one's surroundings. A clean and clutter-free environment fosters a sense of calm, serenity, and vitality, supporting overall well-being.

Reiki Self-Cleansing: Reiki channels universal life force energy to promote relaxation, stress reduction, and holistic healing. Reiki self-cleansing techniques focus on clearing energetic blockages, releasing stagnant energy, and restoring the balance between mind, body, and spirit.

Channeling Healing Energy: Reiki practitioners channel healing energy through their hands to cleanse and balance the chakras (energy centers) and energy fields. By directing Reiki energy towards areas of tension or imbalance, individuals can release energetic blockages and promote the free flow of vital life force energy.

Releasing Mental Clutter: Reiki self-cleansing practices help individuals release mental clutter and negative thought patterns that contribute to stress, anxiety, and being overwhelmed. By connecting with the soothing and transformative energy of Reiki, individuals can let go of mental distractions and experience a sense of clarity, peace, and inner harmony.

Promoting Self-Care Boundaries: Reiki self-cleansing empowers individuals to prioritize self-care boundaries by honoring their need for relaxation, rejuvenation, and spiritual nourishment. By integrating Reiki into their self-care routine, individuals can establish healthy boundaries that protect their physical, emotional, and energetic well-being.

Integration and Practice: By integrating the principles of Saucha and Reiki self-cleansing into our daily lives, individuals can cultivate a deeper sense of purity, clarity, and self-care. Through mindfulness, self-reflection, and intentional energy work, individuals can clear mental clutter, establish boundaries, and prioritize their well-being with greater ease and grace. The combined practice of Saucha and Reiki self-cleansing offers a powerful pathway to inner transformation, personal empowerment, and spiritual evolution.

An Example of How to Use Saucha (Purity) and Reiki Self-Cleansing to Prioritize Self-Care Boundaries

Scenario: Maya is a busy professional and Reiki Practitioner who recognizes the importance of maintaining mental clarity and prioritizing self-care boundaries in her life. Integrating the principle of Saucha from yoga philosophy and Reiki self-cleansing techniques, Maya embarks on a journey to clear mental clutter and cultivate a more profound sense of well-being.

Recognizing the Need for Purity: Maya reflects on her daily life and notices a build-up of mental clutter. She is overwhelmed by her busy schedule and constant multitasking. She realizes that she needs to prioritize self-care and establish boundaries to maintain mental clarity and emotional balance.

Setting Intentions: Maya intends to cultivate purity in her thoughts, emotions, and actions. She affirms her commitment to honoring her well-being and creating space for self-care amidst her busy lifestyle.

Reiki Self-Cleansing Practice: Maya begins her Reiki self-cleansing practice by finding a quiet, peaceful space to relax and center herself. She sits comfortably and closes her eyes, taking a few deep breaths to ground herself in the present moment.

Clearing Energetic Blockages: Maya practices Reiki meditation to channel energy through her body, focusing on areas where she feels tension or blockages. She visualizes the energy flowing freely, clearing away any stagnant or negative energy that may contribute to mental clutter or emotional distress.

Releasing Attachments: As Maya continues her Reiki self-cleansing practice, she consciously releases attachments to thoughts, emotions, or beliefs that no longer serve her highest good. She lets go of perfectionism, self-doubt, and the need for external validation, allowing herself to experience inner peace and acceptance.

Setting Boundaries: With renewed clarity and purity, Maya sets boundaries to protect her mental and emotional well-being. She establishes limits on her workload, prioritizes self-care activities such as meditation and yoga, and communicates her needs to friends and family.

Cultivating Self-Compassion: Maya practices self-compassion and forgiveness, recognizing that setting boundaries is an act of self-love and self-respect. She acknowledges that it's okay to prioritize her well-being and say no to activities or commitments that drain her energy or compromise her boundaries.

Integrating Saucha into Daily Life: Maya integrates the principle of Saucha into her daily life by practicing mindfulness, engaging in activities that bring her joy and fulfillment, and maintaining a balance between work and leisure. She prioritizes self-care boundaries and honors her need for rest and rejuvenation.

By integrating Saucha from yoga philosophy and Reiki self-cleansing techniques, Maya experiences a profound transformation in her ability to clear mental clutter, prioritize self-care, and establish boundaries that honor her well-being. She embraces a life of greater balance, clarity, and inner peace.

An Example of How to Use Saucha to Clear Mental Clutter

Scenario: Liam, a dedicated professional, is often overwhelmed by the mental clutter accumulated from his demanding job and busy lifestyle. Recognizing the need to prioritize self-care and establish boundaries, Liam turns to the Saucha principle from yoga philosophy. He explores alternative meditation techniques to clear his mind and nurture his well-being.

Acknowledging the Need for Purity: Liam reflects on his daily experiences and acknowledges the mental clutter that weighs him down. He realizes he must create space for clarity and inner peace by prioritizing self-care boundaries.

Setting Intentions: With a clear intention to cultivate purity in his thoughts and actions, Liam commits to incorporating Saucha principles into his daily life. He affirms his dedication to nurturing his mental and emotional well-being.

Exploring Alternative Meditation Practices: While Liam is not a Reiki practitioner, he recognizes the value of alternative meditation practices for releasing tension in his mind. He explores mindfulness techniques, such as breath awareness or body scan meditation, to calm his thoughts and clear mental clutter.

Mindfulness Meditation Practice: Liam begins his mindfulness meditation practice by finding a quiet and comfortable space where he can sit undisturbed. He focuses on his breath, observing the natural rhythm of inhalation and exhalation.

Breath Awareness: Liam directs his attention to the sensation of air flowing in and out of his nostrils. With each inhale and exhale, he gently guides his awareness to the present moment, letting go of distractions and worries.

Body Scan: Liam performs a body scan, systematically bringing awareness to each part of his body, from head to toe. He notices any tension or discomfort and consciously releases the tension with each exhale, allowing his body to relax and unwind.

Releasing Mental Clutter: Liam cultivates a sense of spaciousness and clarity through mindfulness meditation. He observes his thoughts with detached awareness, letting go of mental clutter and returning to the present moment with each breath.

Establishing Boundaries: With a renewed sense of purity and clarity, Liam sets boundaries to protect his mental and emotional well-being. He establishes limits on his workload, prioritizes self-care activities, and communicates his needs assertively.

Cultivating Self-Compassion: Liam practices self-compassion and kindness towards himself, recognizing that setting boundaries is an act of self-love and self-respect. He embraces the importance of prioritizing his well-being without guilt or hesitation.

Integrating Saucha into Daily Life: Liam integrates the principle of Saucha into his daily routine by incorporating mindfulness practices, such as meditation and gentle movement, into his schedule. He creates moments of stillness and presence amidst the busyness of life, fostering a sense of purity and inner peace.

Through exploring alternative meditation practices and applying Saucha principles, Liam experiences a profound shift in his ability to clear mental clutter, establish boundaries, and prioritize self-care. He embraces a life of greater balance, clarity, and well-being, guided by purity and inner harmony.

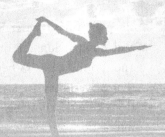

CHAPTER 12

Boundaries with Santosha (Contentment) and Reiki Gratitude

Let's explore how the concepts of Santosha (Contentment) and Reiki Gratitude relate to healthy boundary formation.

Santosha (Contentment)

Acceptance of Self: Santosha encourages individuals to accept themselves as they are without needing external validation or approval. This self-acceptance forms the foundation for healthy boundaries as individuals learn to honor and respect their needs, values, and limits.

Clarity of Priorities: Contentment with one's current circumstances allows individuals to clarify their priorities and what truly matters to them. This clarity enables individuals to set boundaries that align with their values and goals, helping them focus on what is essential and meaningful in their lives.

Respect for Others: Santosha fosters a sense of respect and compassion for others, recognizing their autonomy and boundaries. When individuals are content within themselves, they are less likely to seek validation or control from others, allowing for healthier and more respectful interactions.

Reiki Gratitude

Gratitude for Self-Care: Reiki Gratitude encourages individuals to express gratitude for the self-care practices that nurture their physical, emotional, and spiritual well-being. Individuals can establish boundaries that protect their health and vitality by prioritizing self-care and honoring their needs.

Appreciation for Boundaries: Practicing gratitude for the boundaries set by oneself and others fosters a deeper appreciation for the importance of healthy boundaries in relationships. Individuals recognize that boundaries are essential for maintaining respect, trust, and balance in relationships, leading to greater harmony and mutual understanding.

Alignment with Universal Flow: Reiki Gratitude aligns individuals with the universal flow of energy and abundance, promoting a sense of interconnectedness and unity with all creation. This alignment empowers individuals to set boundaries from a place of self-assurance and trust in the natural order of life, fostering resilience and empowerment.

Integration and Practice: By integrating the principles of Santosha and Reiki Gratitude into their boundary-setting process, individuals can cultivate a more profound sense of self-awareness, compassion, and respect for themselves and others. Through mindfulness, gratitude practices, and intentional energy work, individuals can establish boundaries that honor their well-being and promote healthy, balanced relationships. The combined practice of Santosha and Reiki Gratitude provides a holistic approach to boundary formation, fostering a sense of inner peace, empowerment, and fulfillment in all aspects of life.

An Example of How Santosha (Contentment) and Reiki Gratitude Create Healthy Boundaries

Scenario: Monica, a wife and mother, has been feeling overwhelmed by the demands of her job and family responsibilities. She often finds herself sacrificing her own needs and boundaries to accommodate the needs of others, leading to feelings of resentment and burnout. Recognizing the importance of setting healthy boundaries, Monica integrates the principles of Santosha and Reiki Gratitude into her boundary-setting process.

Santosha (Contentment)

Acceptance of Self: Monica begins by practicing self-acceptance and recognizing her worth and value independent of external validation. She acknowledges that it's okay to prioritize her well-being and set boundaries that honor her needs and limits.

Clarity of Priorities: Through reflection and introspection, Monica clarifies her priorities and what matters most. She identifies the areas where she needs to establish boundaries to protect her physical, emotional, and mental health.

Respect for Others: Santosha fosters a sense of respect and compassion for others, including Monica's family members. She understands that setting boundaries is not about controlling others but respecting their autonomy and creating healthy dynamics in relationships.

Reiki Gratitude

Gratitude for Self-Care: Monica expresses gratitude for the self-care practices that nurture her well-being, such as meditation, exercise, and spending quality time with loved ones. She recognizes that prioritizing self-care is essential for maintaining balance and resilience.

Appreciation for Boundaries: Monica acknowledges the importance of boundaries in relationships and expresses gratitude for the boundaries set by herself and others. She understands that boundaries create a framework for healthy communication, mutual respect, and emotional safety.

Alignment with Universal Flow: Through Reiki Gratitude, Monica aligns herself with the universal flow of energy and abundance. She trusts in the natural order of life and feels empowered to set boundaries from a place of self-assurance and inner peace.

Outcome: With a deeper understanding of Santosha and Reiki Gratitude, Monica begins implementing healthy boundaries in her life. She communicates her needs and limits to her family members with honesty and compassion, fostering open dialogue and mutual understanding. Monica prioritizes self-care activities and makes time for rest, relaxation, and rejuvenation. She recognizes that she can become a better partner, parent, and individual by caring for herself. As Monica practices Santosha and Reiki Gratitude daily, she experiences a profound shift in her relationships and overall well-being. She feels more empowered, fulfilled, and connected to herself and others, knowing she is honoring her boundaries and living authentically.

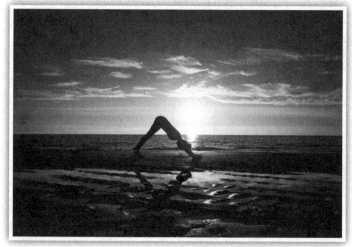

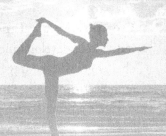

CHAPTER 13

Boundaries with Tapas (Discipline) and Reiki Practice

Tapas, one of the Niyamas (personal observances) in yoga philosophy, refers to self-discipline, austerity, and commitment to one's spiritual and personal growth. It involves cultivating strength, resilience, and determination to overcome obstacles and achieve goals.

Commitment to Personal Growth: Tapas encourages individuals to commit to their personal growth and well-being, even when faced with challenges or discomfort. It requires dedication and perseverance in cultivating positive habits and letting go of unhealthy patterns.

Self-Regulation and Control: Tapas involves self-regulation and control over one's thoughts, emotions, and actions. It empowers individuals to make conscious choices that align with their values and intentions rather than succumbing to impulses or external pressures.

Cultivation of Inner Strength: Through Tapas, individuals develop inner strength and resilience to face life's challenges with courage and equanimity. It fosters a sense of empowerment and self-confidence, enabling individuals to navigate adversity with grace and composure.

Reiki Practice: Reiki as a technique promotes relaxation, stress reduction, and holistic healing. Reiki practice can complement Tapas by providing a supportive framework for self-care, energy balancing, and boundary setting.

Self-Care and Energetic Balance: Reiki practice encourages individuals to prioritize self-care and energetic balance by incorporating regular self-treatments into daily routines. Through Reiki self-treatment, individuals can release tension, restore harmony, and replenish their energy reserves, fostering a sense of well-being and vitality.

Clearing Energetic Blockages: Reiki helps individuals identify and clear energetic blockages that may hinder their personal growth or cause imbalance. By channeling Reiki energy to areas of tension or stagnation, individuals can release old patterns, traumas, and limiting beliefs, paving the way for greater clarity and freedom.

Setting Energetic Boundaries: Reiki empowers individuals to set energetic boundaries to protect their personal space and well-being. By visualizing and reinforcing energetic shields or barriers, individuals can create a sense of safety and security, preventing energetic drains or intrusions from others.

Integration and Practice: By integrating Tapas and Reiki practice, individuals can cultivate a holistic approach to finding peace and setting boundaries around their personal needs:

Commitment to Self-Care: Individuals prioritize self-care and well-being as essential to their daily routine. They incorporate Reiki self-treatment, meditation, yoga, and mindfulness to nurture their body, mind, and spirit.

Self-Discipline and Consistency: Individuals cultivate self-discipline and consistency in their Reiki practice, committing to regular self-treatments and energy maintenance rituals. They set aside time each day or week to engage in Reiki practice, honoring their commitment to personal growth and energetic balance.

Boundary Setting and Self-Protection: Individuals use Reiki practice to set energetic boundaries and protect their personal space from external influences or energies. They can visualize themselves surrounded by a bubble of Reiki energy or use specific Reiki techniques to reinforce their boundaries and shield themselves from negativity or intrusion.

Inner Strength and Resilience: Through the combined practice of Tapas and Reiki, individuals develop inner strength and resilience to face life's challenges with grace and equanimity. They cultivate a sense of empowerment and self-confidence, knowing they have the tools and resources to navigate adversity and maintain their well-being.

Peace and Harmony: Ultimately, integrating Tapas and Reiki practice leads to greater peace, harmony, and balance in individuals' lives. They experience a deep sense of inner peace and contentment, knowing that they are honoring their needs and boundaries while fostering spiritual and energetic growth.

By embracing Tapas and Reiki practice as complementary tools for personal transformation and boundary setting, individuals can cultivate a deeper connection to themselves, others, and the world around them, leading to a life of greater peace, fulfillment, and well-being.

An Example of How to Cultivate Discipline to Uphold Boundaries Aligned with Your Inner Values

Scenario: Luke is a software engineer who works long hours at a demanding tech company. He often feels stressed, exhausted, and overwhelmed by the pressures of his job. Additionally, Luke struggles with setting boundaries in his personal life, frequently saying yes to requests and obligations that drain his energy and leave him feeling depleted. Recognizing the need for change, Luke integrates Tapas (Discipline) and Reiki meditation into his daily routine to prioritize self-care and establish healthy boundaries.

Commitment to Self-Care (Tapas)

Creating a Self-Care Routine: Luke commits to creating a self-care routine that includes daily practices to nurture his physical, emotional, and spiritual well-being. He sets aside time each morning for meditation, Reiki self-treatment, and gentle yoga to start his day on a positive note.

Setting Work-Life Boundaries: Luke establishes clear boundaries between his work and personal life, committing to disconnecting from work emails and notifications outside of office hours. He prioritizes activities that bring him joy and relaxation, such as spending time with loved ones, pursuing hobbies, and enjoying nature.

Self-Discipline and Consistency (Tapas)

Sticking to a Schedule: Luke practices self-discipline by following a consistent schedule for his self-care practices and boundary-setting activities. He sets alarms or reminders on his phone to ensure he takes regular daily breaks to rest and recharge.

Accountability and Tracking Progress: Luke holds himself accountable for his commitments to self-care and boundary-setting by tracking his progress in a journal. He reflects on his achievements and challenges, celebrating successes and adjusting his approach.

Boundary Setting and Self-Protection (Reiki Meditation)

Energetic Boundaries: Luke uses Reiki meditation to visualize and reinforce energetic boundaries around himself, particularly in high-stress or challenging situations at work. He visualizes peaceful Reiki energy surrounding him, deflecting negativity and preserving his inner peace.

Saying No with Compassion: Luke learns to say no to requests and obligations that do not align with his priorities or values, using Reiki principles of compassion and empathy. He communicates his boundaries assertively yet kindly, honoring his own needs while respecting the needs of others.

Inner Strength and Resilience (Tapas and Reiki Meditation)

Building Inner Strength: Through the combined practice of Tapas and Reiki meditation, Luke builds inner strength and resilience to navigate the challenges of his job and personal life with grace and equanimity. He cultivates a sense of empowerment and self-confidence, knowing he has the tools to overcome obstacles and maintain his well-being.

Releasing Stress and Tension: Luke uses Reiki meditation to release stress, tension, and emotional baggage accumulated throughout the day. He meditates to clear stagnant energy and restore balance, allowing him to approach each new day with renewed vitality and clarity.

Outcome: As Luke integrates Tapas and Reiki meditation into his daily life, he experiences a profound transformation in his overall well-being and quality of life. He feels more grounded, centered, and at peace with himself and his surroundings. By prioritizing self-care and setting boundaries around his personal needs, Luke creates a more balanced, fulfilling life aligned with his true essence. He navigates challenges with resilience and grace, knowing he has the strength and resources to thrive in any situation.

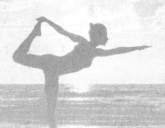

CHAPTER 14

Boundaries with Svadhyaya (Self-Study) and Reiki Self-Reflection

Svadhyaya, one of the Niyamas in the Eight Limbs of Yoga, is often translated as "self-study." However, this practice extends beyond merely introspecting on our thoughts and actions; it includes the study of external sources, traditionally sacred texts, to deepen our understanding of ourselves and the world around us.

Studying external sources keeps us humble and curious, reminding us that we are ever-evolving beings who can continually learn and grow. By approaching ourselves as study subjects—rather than assuming we already fully understand who we are—we open ourselves to new insights and perspectives. This mindset fosters a sense of humility as we recognize that we are part of a larger whole, reflecting the world in a microcosm. Every interaction and experience thus becomes an opportunity for self-learning and growth.

Exploration of Inner Landscape: Svadhyaya encourages individuals to explore their inner landscape with curiosity and openness. Through self-study, individuals gain insight into their thought patterns, emotional triggers, and underlying motivations, allowing them to identify areas where boundaries may need to be established or reinforced.

Awareness of Limiting Beliefs: Self-study helps individuals become aware of limiting beliefs or self-imposed limitations that may hinder their ability to set healthy boundaries. By examining the stories they tell themselves and challenging outdated beliefs, individuals can cultivate a greater sense of self-worth and empowerment, laying the foundation for assertive boundary-setting.

Alignment with Authentic Self: Svadhyaya invites individuals to align with their authentic self and core values. Through self-reflection, individuals gain clarity about what is truly important to them and where to draw boundaries to honor their integrity, well-being, and personal growth journey.

Reiki Self-Reflection complements this aspect of Svadhyaya by encouraging us to connect with our energy on a deeper level. Through Reiki, we can observe how external influences affect our energetic state and how our internal landscape mirrors the world around us. Just as Svadhyaya invites us to explore sacred texts, Reiki invites us to explore the sacred text of our energy, learning to read and understand it with clarity and compassion.

Reiki Self-Reflection: Reiki Self-Reflection involves using Reiki principles and energy work techniques to explore and address energetic imbalances, emotional patterns, and subconscious beliefs that may impact boundary-setting and interpersonal dynamics.

Energetic Awareness: Reiki Self-Reflection enhances energetic awareness, allowing individuals to tune into their subtle energy body and detect areas of congestion, depletion, or imbalance. By scanning their energy field, individuals can identify where energetic boundaries may be weak or compromised, signaling the need for self-care and boundary reinforcement.

Emotional Release: Reiki Self-Reflection facilitates the release of pent-up emotions, traumas, and unresolved issues that may influence boundary-setting patterns. Through Reiki treatments or self-healing sessions, individuals can release emotional baggage and create space for healthier boundaries to emerge, free from past conditioning or attachments.

Clarity and Intuition: Reiki Self-Reflection enhances clarity and intuition, allowing individuals to discern their actual needs, desires, and boundaries with greater accuracy. Individuals can set boundaries aligned with their highest good and soul's purpose by connecting to their inner guidance system and trusting their intuitive insights.

By integrating Svadhyaya and Reiki Self-Reflection into our lives, we create a dynamic practice of inward and outward-looking self-study. This balanced approach helps us set healthy boundaries as we better understand our needs and limitations and how they interact with the world around us. Each moment becomes an opportunity to learn, grow, and refine the boundaries that support our well-being and personal growth.

An Example of How to Integrate Svadhyaya and Reiki Self-Reflection

Scenario: Krista, a busy professional and mother of two, often feels overwhelmed by the demands placed on her by work, family, and friends. She frequently says "yes" to requests, leaving little time for herself, and this pattern has left her feeling depleted and resentful. Recognizing the need to set more explicit boundaries, Krista turns to Svadhyaya, or self-study, as a guiding principle in her journey toward balance.

Reflecting on Values and Priorities: Krista begins by reflecting deeply on her core values and priorities. She journals about what matters most to her—her career aspirations, relationships, and self-care needs. This self-study process helps her clarify the areas in her life where boundaries are essential to honor her values and maintain a healthy balance.

Exploration of Emotional Triggers: As part of her self-study, Krista examines her emotional triggers and behavior patterns that lead her to overextend herself. She reflects on past experiences where she felt resentful or exhausted due to a lack of boundaries. By gaining insight into these triggers, Krista becomes more aware of situations where she is likely to compromise her well-being. This awareness allows her to anticipate and prepare for such situations, making boundary-setting a more proactive and conscious practice.

Identification of Limiting Beliefs: Krista also identifies limiting beliefs that may hold her from setting assertive boundaries. She notices thoughts like, "I have to say yes for them to like me" or "I don't want to let them down," contributing to her overcommitment. Through Svadhyaya, Krista challenges these beliefs and reframes them with more empowering ones, such as "Setting boundaries is an act of self-respect and self-care." This shift in mindset enables her to approach boundary-setting with greater confidence and self-assurance.

External Study and Humility: Krista turns to external sources for guidance in addition to her internal reflections. She reads about boundary-setting and self-care in yoga philosophy, self-help books, and spiritual teachings. These resources provide her with new perspectives, helping her understand that her challenges are not unique but are part of a broader human experience. This external study keeps Krista humble and curious, reminding her that self-study is an ongoing process of learning and growth.

Reiki Self-Reflection: Krista incorporates Reiki Self-Reflection into her daily routine, tuning into her energy to observe how different situations and interactions affect her. She notices that her energy feels scattered and drained when she agrees to something out of guilt or obligation. Conversely, her energy feels more grounded and clear when she honors her needs and sets boundaries. Reiki helps Krista reinforce the connection between her internal state and her external actions, guiding her toward healthier, more sustainable practices.

Holistic Integration: Through this combined practice of Svadhyaya and Reiki, Krista sees boundary-setting as a task and a holistic practice that honors her well-being and her place in the larger world. She understands that setting boundaries is not only about protecting her energy but also about creating healthier dynamics in her relationships. This approach allows Krista to set boundaries with compassion and confidence, knowing she fosters a more balanced and harmonious life.

By integrating the principles of the Eight Limbs of Yoga and the reflective practices of Reiki, we've seen how boundaries can become more than just lines of defense—they can be expressions of self-respect, compassion, and balance. Through Svadhyaya (self-study), we gain awareness and understand our needs and limits. At the same time, Reiki helps us attune to our energy, ensuring that our boundaries support our overall well-being.

Setting boundaries is not about isolation or exclusion; it's about creating the space for authentic connection with ourselves and others. As we've seen in the scenarios, this process is dynamic and requires continuous reflection and adjustment. It's about learning to say "no" with kindness, navigating relationships with integrity, and finding the balance that honors our true selves.

As you continue on your journey, remember that boundary-setting is a practice, much like yoga and Reiki. It evolves as you do, and with each step, you strengthen your ability to live in alignment with your highest values. Embrace this process with patience and compassion, knowing that every boundary you set is a step toward a more harmonious and empowered life.

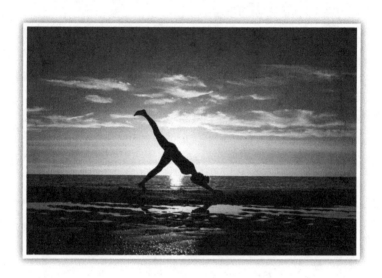

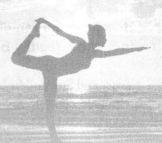

CHAPTER 15

Boundaries with Ishvara Pranidhana (Surrender to a Higher Power) and Reiki

Ishvara Pranidhana, one of the Niyamas in the eight limbs of yoga, translates to surrender to a higher power. It encourages us to trust the universe and let go of the ego's need for control. This principle fosters humility, acceptance, and a sense of peace, allowing us to flow with life's changes rather than resisting them.

Reiki, a practice centered on channeling universal life force energy for healing, aligns beautifully with Ishvara Pranidhana. Reiki practitioners trust in the universal energy to guide the healing process, surrendering control and allowing the energy to flow where it is needed most. This surrender enhances the practitioner's ability to maintain a balanced and harmonious energy state.

How Ishvara Pranidhana and Reiki Aid in Setting Healthy Boundaries

Trust and Surrender: Ishvara Pranidhana teaches us to trust in a higher power and surrender control. This trust enables us to set boundaries without fear or anxiety, knowing that the universe supports us.

Letting Go of Control: Both Ishvara Pranidhana and Reiki emphasize letting go of the need to control every aspect of our lives. This release allows us to establish boundaries that prioritize our well-being over the demands and expectations of others.

Enhanced Intuition: Reiki practice heightens our intuition, helping us to sense when our boundaries are being crossed and when adjustments are needed. This intuitive guidance aligns with surrendering to a higher power, providing a clear path to maintaining healthy boundaries.

Inner Peace: The surrender aspect of Ishvara Pranidhana and the healing energy of Reiki foster inner peace. This calm state of mind is crucial for confidently setting and enforcing boundaries without emotional turmoil.

An Example of How to Use Ishvara Pranidhana and Reiki at Work and Home

Scenario: Kelly is a dedicated therapist who balances her demanding job with raising a family. She has a husband and three children aged 15, 9, and 3. Despite her best efforts, she often finds herself overwhelmed, struggling to set boundaries between her professional and personal life.

Recognizing the Need for Surrender: Kelly acknowledges her need to control every aspect of her life and the resulting stress. She embraces Ishvara Pranidhana, trusting she can create a healthier balance by letting go.

Reiki Self-Healing: Kelly starts practicing Reiki self-healing to release the accumulated stress and to realign her energy. She uses Reiki meditative practices to channel universal energy, promoting relaxation and clarity.

Setting Boundaries with Trust: With renewed trust in the universe, Kelly sets clear boundaries for her work and personal life. She decides not to take work calls after a particular hour and schedules specific times for family activities, trusting that her practice will flourish without constant overextension. Kelly shares responsibilities with her husband and children and trusts them to show up the best they can. Kelly releases her expectations of how things "should" be and accepts the present as a gift.

Communicating Boundaries: Kelly communicates these boundaries to her clients and family, explaining the importance of maintaining a healthy balance. She reassures her clients that their sessions will be more effective when she is well-rested and focused.

Practicing Consistent Surrender: Kelly incorporates daily practices of Ishvara Pranidhana and Reiki, reinforcing her boundaries and maintaining her inner peace. She finds that she can effectively manage her roles as a therapist and mother by surrendering control and trusting in the universal flow.

Ishvara Pranidhana and Reiki offer profound insights and tools for setting healthy boundaries. By trusting in a higher power and surrendering the need for control, we can establish boundaries that honor our well-being and create a harmonious balance. These practices encourage us to live with intention, clarity, and peace, making boundary-setting a natural and essential part of our journey.

CHAPTER 16

Boundaries in Relations through Asanas (Poses) and Reiki Healing

Cultivating healthy boundaries is paramount in personal growth, well-being, and especially within relationships. Boundaries serve as essential guidelines defining our physical, emotional, and energetic limits, allowing us to honor our needs, values, and autonomy while fostering mutual respect and understanding. In the fusion of ancient practices like yoga and Reiki Healing, we discover powerful tools to deepen our self-awareness and fortify our ability to establish and maintain boundaries. The third limb of yoga is Asana or yoga poses. Through the harmonious integration of Asana, which promotes physical strength and inner stability, and Reiki Healing techniques, which facilitate energetic balance and self-nurturing, individuals can navigate relationships with grace, clarity, and authenticity. Let us embark on a journey into the synergy of yoga and Reiki, exploring how these practices can empower us to cultivate healthy boundaries and harmonious connections.

Standing Poses and Reiki Grounding: Standing poses, such as Warrior and Mountain Pose, establish a strong foundation, promoting energetic grounding and stability. These poses symbolize the need for firm boundaries, creating a sense of rootedness that reflects our inner strength. Integrating Reiki grounding techniques during these poses can enhance the feeling of being centered and secure.

Balancing Poses and Reiki Harmony: Balancing poses, like Tree Pose or Eagle Pose, challenge our physical equilibrium and reflect the importance of maintaining balance in relationships. Incorporating Reiki harmony techniques can enhance our ability to stay centered and calm, even in interpersonal dynamics.

Seated Poses and Reiki Communication: Seated poses such as Lotus or Seated Forward Bend encourage introspection and communication with oneself. Reiki can aid in clearing energetic blockages and promoting clear expression of boundaries. These poses help cultivate stability in communication, allowing us to assert our needs and limits effectively.

Restorative Poses and Reiki Self-Nurturing: Restorative poses, such as Child's Pose or Legs-Up-The-Wall Pose, offer deep relaxation and self-nurturing. They are crucial for understanding and honoring our boundaries by providing time for self-care and regeneration. Reiki self-nurturing practices during these poses support emotional and physical healing, reinforcing the importance of self-care in maintaining healthy boundaries.

Using Props in Asana Practice: Props, such as blocks, straps, and bolsters, play a significant role in enhancing our asana practice. They shift the aim from merely attaining or performing the pose to creating an experience that encourages a deeper focus on one's inner experience. By using props, we can rely on our surroundings and resources, acknowledging our physical limits and the extent to which we can explore and expand our boundaries with what is available. Props help deepen the time and intensity in a pose, allowing for a more profound experience of stability, balance, and self-nurturing. They support us in cultivating an awareness of our boundaries and adjusting our practice to meet our personal needs and capacities.

Integrating asanas, Reiki, and boundary-setting offers a comprehensive approach to fostering balance and clarity in our lives. By aligning physical practices with energetic principles, we create a harmonious environment that supports establishing and maintaining healthy boundaries. Standing and balancing poses ground us and promote stability, while restorative poses and Reiki self-nurturing provide essential space for self-care and healing. The mindful use of props enhances our practice, encouraging deeper self-awareness and adaptation to our needs. This holistic approach strengthens our physical and energetic boundaries and nurtures our overall well-being, enabling us to navigate relationships and interactions with greater confidence and compassion.

An Example of Enhanced Yoga Practice for Boundary Setting

Scenario: Having recently addressed her boundary-setting challenges with Alex's help and sought new resources, Jamie is now committed to integrating these insights into her yoga practice. After first consulting her physician, she decided to try yoga to help release built-up energy and reinforce her boundaries. She discovers a dynamic sequence that includes vinyasa flow, strategic use of props, and a focus on self-care.

Jamie's practice begins with a grounding approach and transitions into a more dynamic flow to invigorate her body and mind.

Warm-Up and Grounding:

Mountain Pose (Tadasana): Jamie starts in Mountain Pose to establish stability and alignment, connecting with the ground beneath her.

Vinyasa Flow:

Forward Fold (Uttanasana): Jamie begins with Forward Fold, using a chair as a prop to support her back and create space as she folds forward. This modification helps alleviate strain and allows her to focus on deepening her breath and relaxation.

Sun Salutation A: She moves into Sun Salutation A, incorporating Downward Dog and Plank Pose to engage her entire body and elevate her heart rate. A couple rounds of this flow helps prepare her for more dynamic movement.

Sun Salutation B: Jamie then transitions into Sun Salutation B, adding Chair Pose and Warrior I to engage her core and legs further. This sequence builds strength and prepares her for the more challenging poses ahead.

Pose Sequence with Props:

Tree Pose (Vrksasana): Jamie practices Tree Pose with a block under her lifted foot for additional stability. This adjustment allows her to focus on rooting down through the standing leg while finding balance and alignment.

Warrior II (Virabhadrasana II): She incorporates Warrior II to cultivate inner strength and resilience, maintaining focus and balance.

Forward Fold (Uttanasana) Again: Returning to Forward Fold, Jamie uses the chair prop again, if needed for support, to release any residual tension and deepen her stretch.

Restorative Poses:

Child's Pose (Balasana): Jamie moves into Child's Pose as needed for rest and integration, using a blanket under her knees for added comfort. This restorative pose helps her reconnect with her inner self and integrate her practice.

Savasana (Corpse Pose): Jamie concludes her practice with Savasana, focusing on complete relaxation and absorption of the benefits of her practice. She uses a bolster or blanket to support her body and promote deep, restorative relaxation.

Yoga in an asana practice offers profound benefits beyond physical fitness, supporting mental and energetic well-being. Moving mindfully through each posture releases physical tension, quiets mental chatter, and clears emotional blockages, cultivating awareness and resilience. This foundation supports healthy boundaries by helping us recognize what serves us and release what doesn't.

Reiki and more profound meditation further enrich this journey, addressing the subtle energy layers that shape our interactions. Reiki brings healing energy to clear and balance our essence, while deep meditation strengthens our self-connection, providing insight from a calm, focused state. Yoga, Reiki, and meditation foster a balanced, centered life that radiates outward, enriching our relationships and creating harmony in our surroundings. Through these practices, we discover peace, clarity, and the wisdom to engage in mindful, loving connections.

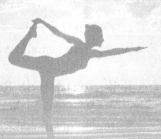

CHAPTER 17

Self-Care and Social Boundaries with Pranayama and Reiki Energy Work

Let's dig into honoring self-care boundaries for emotional well-being and navigating social boundaries with Pranayama (breath work) and Reiki Energy Work. Pranayama, or breath control, is a yoga practice that involves regulating the breath to enhance the flow of vital energy, or prana, throughout the body. It promotes self-awareness, emotional balance, and mental clarity. Reiki energy work provides deep relaxation by channeling universal life force energy to promote healing and balance on physical, emotional, mental, and spiritual levels. Pranayama and Reiki provide powerful tools for honoring self-care boundaries and navigating social interactions with clarity and compassion.

Honoring Self-Care Boundaries for Emotional Well-Being

Breath Awareness: Cultivating awareness of the breath is fundamental in yoga and Reiki practice. By paying attention to the breath, individuals can anchor themselves in the present moment and connect with their inner state.

Reiki Breathwork: Reiki Breathwork involves using the breath to channel healing energy throughout the body. Through intentional breathing techniques, individuals can release emotional tension, restore balance, and promote relaxation in both body and mind.

Social Boundaries with Pranayama and Reiki Energy Work

Equal Breathing: Equal Breathing, where the inhalation and exhalation are of equal length, promotes balance and harmony in the body and mind. It fosters a sense of equanimity and stability, which is essential for navigating social boundaries.

Reiki Exchange: Reiki Exchange involves individuals' mutual giving and receiving of healing energy. By establishing clear boundaries around energy exchange, individuals can maintain equilibrium in relationships and prevent energetic depletion or imbalance.

Nadi Shodhana: Nadi Shodhana, or Alternate Nostril Breathing, is a Pranayama technique that balances energy flow through the body's subtle energy channels (nadis). It promotes mental clarity, emotional balance, and harmonious energy flow.

Reiki Flow: Reiki Flow refers to the natural movement of healing energy through the practitioner and recipient during a Reiki session. By harmonizing boundaries with compassion and empathy, Reiki practitioners can facilitate a smooth and nurturing flow of energy that supports healing and well-being.

Integration of Practices

Using Breath to Establish Energetic Boundaries: Individuals can use breath awareness and intentional breathing techniques to establish energetic boundaries in social interactions. They can maintain inner stability and clarity while navigating interpersonal dynamics by centering themselves in the breath.

Balancing Giving and Receiving Energy: Through practices like Equal Breathing and Reiki Exchange, individuals can cultivate balance and reciprocity in relationships. They can set boundaries around energy exchange to ensure that their needs for replenishment and self-care are honored.

Harmonizing Boundaries with Compassion: Nadi Shodhana and Reiki Flow encourage individuals to approach boundary-setting with compassion and empathy. By harmonizing boundaries with the flow of universal life force energy, individuals can foster deeper connections and understanding in their relationships.

In summary, honoring self-care boundaries for emotional well-being and navigating social boundaries with

Pranayama and Reiki Energy Work involves integrating breath awareness, intentional breathing techniques, and compassionate boundary-setting practices. By establishing clear boundaries around energy exchange and harmonizing boundaries with empathy, individuals can cultivate healthier and more fulfilling relationships while prioritizing their well-being, leading to greater personal empowerment and energetic balance.

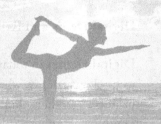

CHAPTER 18

Boundaries with Pratyahara (Withdrawal of the Senses) and Reiki Mindfulness

Let's explore how to cultivate mindfulness and boundaries through Pratyahara (withdrawal of the senses) and Reiki Mindfulness, focusing on sensory awareness, digital detox, and creating sacred space.

Sensory Awareness and Reiki Sensitivity

Sensory Awareness: Pratyahara involves withdrawing the senses from external stimuli and turning inward. Individuals can become more attuned to energetic triggers and their effects on their well-being by cultivating sensory awareness.

Reiki Sensitivity: Reiki mindfulness encourages individuals to cultivate sensitivity to subtle energy shifts within themselves and their environment. Heightened awareness allows individuals to recognize energetic triggers and set boundaries for energetic protection.

Digital Detox and Reiki Self-Care

Digital Detox: In today's digital age, constant exposure to technology can overwhelm the senses and disrupt energetic balance. Practicing Pratyahara involves setting boundaries around technology use and taking regular breaks from screens to restore energetic clarity.

Reiki Self-Care: Reiki self-care techniques, such as self-treatments and energy-clearing practices, help individuals cleanse and rejuvenate their energy fields. By establishing boundaries around technology and prioritizing self-care, individuals can maintain energetic balance and well-being.

Creating Sacred Space and Reiki Energetic Boundaries

Creating Sacred Space: Designating physical spaces for mindfulness practice and boundary-setting fosters a sense of sacredness and intentionality. Whether a meditation corner at home or a quiet outdoor sanctuary, sacred spaces provide a conducive environment for energetic self-reflection.

Reiki Energetic Boundaries: Reiki practitioners often use intention to create energetic boundaries for protection and clarity. Individuals can establish boundaries that support their spiritual and energetic well-being by infusing their surroundings with Reiki energy and setting clear intentions.

Integration of Practices

Noticing Energetic Triggers: Individuals can see when external stimuli or energetic interactions trigger discomfort or imbalance through sensory awareness and Reiki sensitivity. This awareness enables them to set boundaries to protect their energy and maintain inner harmony.

Establishing Boundaries around Technology: By practicing digital detox and Reiki self-care, individuals can create boundaries around technology use to prevent energetic overwhelm and maintain clarity of mind. Setting limits on screen time and incorporating self-care practices promote balance and well-being.

Designating Spaces for Boundary-Setting: Creating sacred space and Reiki energetic boundaries allows individuals to establish a supportive environment for mindfulness practice and energetic self-reflection. These designated spaces serve as reminders to honor boundaries and prioritize self-care in daily life.

In summary, cultivating mindfulness and boundaries through Pratyahara and Reiki Mindfulness involves developing sensory awareness, practicing digital detox, and creating sacred spaces for energetic self-reflection. By integrating these practices into daily life, individuals can enhance their ability to recognize and honor their boundaries, fostering greater clarity, balance, and well-being on all levels.

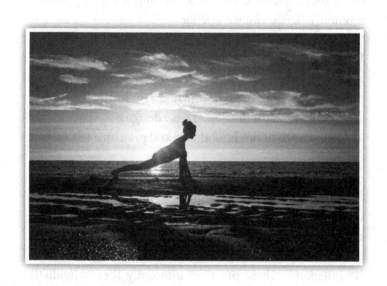

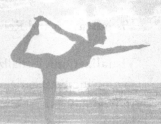

CHAPTER 19

Boundaries through Dharana (Concentration) and Reiki Intent

Let's delve deeper into strengthening boundaries through Dharana (concentration) and Reiki Intent, focusing on techniques such as focus and intention, visualization, and mantra meditation.

Focus and Intention and Reiki Intent

Focus and Intention: Dharana directs attention and concentration toward a single point or goal. Individuals can channel their energy into maintaining boundaries with clarity and purpose by cultivating focus and intention.

Reiki Intent: Reiki practitioners use intention to direct healing energy towards a specific purpose or outcome. Similarly, individuals can infuse their boundary-setting efforts with Reiki intent, aligning their actions with their highest good and the well-being of all involved.

Visualization and Reiki

Visualization: Visualization is a powerful technique for reinforcing boundaries and manifesting desired outcomes. Individuals can strengthen their resolve and maintain healthy boundaries by mentally picturing themselves surrounded by a protective, energetic shield or boundary.

Reiki: Reiki practitioners often use visualization techniques during healing sessions to facilitate energy flow and promote balance. By incorporating Reiki into their visualization practice, individuals can amplify the effectiveness of their boundary-setting efforts and promote energetic harmony.

Mantra Meditation and Reiki Affirmations

Mantra Meditation: Mantra meditation involves repeating a sacred word or phrase to focus the mind and cultivate inner peace. Individuals can bolster their resolve and overcome challenges with grace by using mantras that affirm their worthiness, strength, and ability to maintain boundaries.

Reiki Affirmations: Reiki affirmations are positive statements that reinforce healing and empowerment. By incorporating Reiki affirmations into daily practice, individuals can uphold energetic boundaries and cultivate inner strength, resilience, and self-confidence.

Integration of Practices

Channeling Energy with Clarity and Purpose: Through focus and intention and Reiki intent, individuals can channel their energy into maintaining boundaries with clarity and purpose. They empower themselves to navigate challenging situations with confidence and integrity by setting clear intentions and upholding boundaries.

Reinforcing Healthy Energetic Boundaries: Visualization and Reiki techniques allow individuals to visualize and strengthen healthy energetic boundaries in various situations. By mentally picturing themselves surrounded by protective energy and affirming their right to set and maintain boundaries, they create a supportive inner environment that promotes resilience and well-being.

Using Affirmations for Inner Strength: Mantra meditation and Reiki affirmations provide individuals with powerful tools for cultivating inner strength and resilience. By repeating positive affirmations that reinforce their worthiness and ability to uphold boundaries, they nurture a sense of self-confidence and empowerment that allows them to protect their energy and well-being assertively.

In summary, strengthening boundaries through Dharana and Reiki Intent involves harnessing the power of focus, intention, visualization, and affirmations to uphold energetic boundaries with clarity, purpose, and inner strength. By integrating these practices into their daily lives, individuals can cultivate resilience, assertiveness, and a deeper connection to their innate capacity for self-care and empowerment.

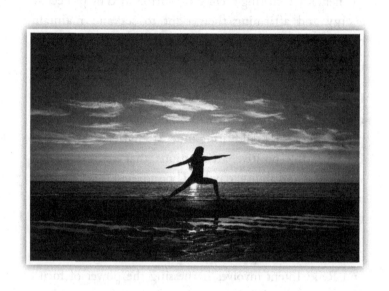

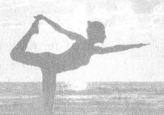

CHAPTER 20

Dhyana (Meditation), Samadhi (Union with the Divine), and Reiki Integration

Meditation is versatile and may be experienced in various forms, from listening to or chanting affirmations to sitting in stillness, walking in nature, or exploring a prayer labyrinth. The key is to discover a meditation style that resonates with and honors who you are. I suggest integrating Reiki with meditation to support energetic alignment in this section. However, proper training and attunement from a certified teacher are essential to genuinely working with Reiki. For more details on Reiki training and resources, visit gotharmony.org.

Dhyana, or meditation, and Samadhi, or union with the divine, are two final stages in Patanjali's Yoga Sutras that guide us towards spiritual liberation. Dhyana involves deep, sustained concentration where the mind becomes fully absorbed in the object of meditation, transcending the distractions of the external world. This continuous flow of attention leads to Samadhi, a state of profound inner stillness and unity, where we experience a dissolution of the ego and a deep connection with the universal consciousness. Together, Dhyana and Samadhi represent the culmination of the yogic path, leading to the ultimate realization of one's true nature.

Dhyana (Meditation) for Boundary Awareness

Purpose: Dhyana, or meditation, allows you to develop a deeper awareness of your internal state, fostering insight into where boundaries are needed. Through focused meditation, you can observe where boundaries are being respected or violated and how this affects your overall well-being.

Practice: Choose a peaceful space and settle into a position that feels comfortable for you. Begin by focusing on your breath and letting go of distractions. As you meditate, reflect on where you feel tension or discomfort—these may be areas where boundaries are lacking or have been crossed. Use this time to explore what boundaries you need to establish to honor your values and maintain balance.

Samadhi (Union with the Divine) for Spiritual Insight into Boundaries

Purpose: Samadhi represents the ultimate dissolution of the ego, where the boundaries between the self and the universe fade away. While this might seem at odds with the concept of setting boundaries, it offers a unique perspective. In Samadhi, you are in complete harmony with the universe's flow beyond the limitations of the ego. This state of union allows you to perceive boundaries not as rigid divisions but as fluid and harmonious expressions of universal balance.

Practice: After a deep meditation session, allow yourself to enter a contemplative state where you release personal concerns and merge with the greater flow of universal energy. In this state, reflect on your boundaries from a place of divine understanding. Recognize that true boundaries are not about separation but about creating a space for the soul to thrive within the larger context of universal harmony. Samadhi can provide insights that transcend intellectual understanding, helping you to intuitively sense which boundaries are in tune with the universe and which are not. It may also help you process complex emotional experiences, such as forgiveness, that are difficult to navigate in everyday life but become clearer in this state of union.

Reiki Integration for Energetic Alignment

Purpose: Reiki complements meditation and the insights gained from Samadhi by providing a practical method to align your energy with the boundaries you've identified. Reiki helps to ensure that your boundaries are not only mentally and emotionally clear but also energetically supported.

Practice: Begin your self-Reiki session by focusing on areas of your body where you feel boundary issues manifest— these could be physical sensations, emotional discomfort, or energy blockages. Use Reiki to balance and clear these areas, visualizing the energy and creating a protective yet flexible boundary around you. Affirm your commitment to maintaining these boundaries in harmony with the universal energy flow, reinforcing the insights gained during your meditation and contemplation.

While Samadhi is the dissolution of boundaries, it offers a profound understanding of them from a place of universal connection. In this state, boundaries are seen not as barriers but as the natural order that allows for harmony and balance in life. By integrating the practices of Dhyana, Samadhi, and Reiki, you can cultivate a deeper awareness of your boundaries, align them with universal truth, and energetically support them in your daily life. This approach not only protects your well-being but also ensures that your boundaries are in tune with the greater flow of life, fostering a balanced and fulfilling existence.

An Example of Rediscovering Connection and Boundaries

Scenario: Chris and Lisa have been married for over 25 years. They recently became empty nesters as their youngest child moved out for college. While they are excited about this new phase of life, they also feel a bit lost and disconnected from each other and themselves. Over the years, their lives revolved around their children, and now they are unsure of how to navigate this new chapter. They want to rediscover their relationship and deepen their connection, both with each other and with their individual selves.

Challenge: As they embark on this journey, Chris and Lisa realize that they need to redefine their personal boundaries and their boundaries as a couple. They've always been a team, but now they need to balance their partnership with their own individual needs and passions. They want to find a way to maintain a strong connection while also exploring new interests and activities independently.

Self-Reflection and Awareness

Lisa's Practice: Lisa begins by dedicating time each morning to self-reflection through journaling and meditation. She explores her feelings about this new phase of life, acknowledging areas where she may have neglected her well-being in the past. She realizes she wants to reconnect with her passion for painting, which she set aside while raising their children.

Chris's Practice: Chris spends time in the evening practicing self-Reiki and meditation, reflecting on his own needs and desires. He recognizes that he has always put others first and now wants to focus on his physical health by returning to his love for hiking and outdoor activities.

Clarifying Boundaries

Couple's Discussion: Chris and Lisa sit down together and discuss their individual needs and goals. They agree that it's essential to support each other's personal growth while also nurturing their relationship. They decide to set specific boundaries around their time, ensuring they each have dedicated time for their individual pursuits without feeling guilty or neglecting their relationship.

Personal Boundaries: Lisa sets a boundary for herself to spend two afternoons a week in her art studio without interruptions. Chris sets a boundary to go hiking every Saturday morning, giving himself space to reconnect with nature.

Communicating Boundaries Clearly

Expressing Needs: Chris and Lisa communicate their boundaries to each other with honesty and respect. Lisa expressed her excitement about getting back into painting and asked Chris to respect her studio time as a sacred space for creativity. Chris shares his desire to explore new hiking trails and asks Lisa to support his need for time outdoors.

Compassionate Communication: They practice using "I" statements to express their feelings and needs, ensuring that their communication is compassionate and understanding. For example, Lisa says, "I feel rejuvenated when I have time to paint, and I'd love your support in keeping that time for myself." Chris responds, "I feel energized when I'm out in nature, and it's important for me to have that time to clear my mind."

Integrating Dhyana, Samadhi, and Reiki

Joint Meditation Practice: To strengthen their connection, Chris and Lisa started a joint meditation practice in the evenings. They sit together in quiet reflection, focusing on their breath and the energy between them. This practice helps them feel more in tune with each other and the universe, fostering a sense of unity and peace.

Reiki Sessions: They also begin exchanging Reiki sessions, using this time to offer each other healing energy and support. Lisa placed her hands over Chris's heart, intending to help him feel grounded and loved, while Chris focused on Lisa's creative energy, helping her feel inspired and free.

Exploring Samadhi: During their meditation, they occasionally enter a deeper state of connection, experiencing moments of Samadhi where they feel completely in tune with each other and the world around them. These experiences help them understand that while their individual boundaries are essential, they are also part of a larger, interconnected whole.

Practicing Self-Care

Individual Activities: Chris and Lisa each engage in activities that nourish their souls. Lisa immerses herself in her art, losing herself in the flow of creativity, while Chris finds joy in challenging hikes and the tranquility of nature.

Couple's Activities: They also make time for activities they enjoy together, such as cooking, dancing, and exploring new places. These shared experiences help them reconnect and rediscover their relationship, building new memories in this new phase of life.

Reflecting and Adjusting

Regular Check-Ins: Chris and Lisa establish a routine of checking in with each other weekly to discuss how they're feeling about their boundaries and their relationship. They use this time to reflect on what's working well and where they might need to make adjustments. This practice helps them stay connected and ensures that their individual needs are met without sacrificing their relationship.

Flexibility and Growth: They remain open to adjusting their boundaries as needed, understanding that this is an ongoing process. They also recognize that as they continue to grow individually, their relationship will evolve, and they are committed to supporting each other through these changes.

Outcome: Through this process, Chris and Lisa rediscover themselves and their relationship. They find a balance between honoring their individual needs and nurturing their connection as a couple. By setting clear boundaries, practicing open communication, and integrating meditation, Samadhi, and Reiki into their lives, they create a harmonious and fulfilling relationship that supports both their personal growth and their love for each other.

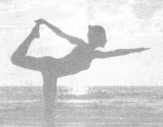

CHAPTER 21

Establishing Boundaries to Maintain Energetic Balance

Establishing boundaries is essential for maintaining energetic balance, allowing individuals to protect their energy, honor their needs, and cultivate a sense of inner harmony. Reiki, complements this practice by emphasizing the harmonious flow of energy within the body and the environment. By integrating Reiki into daily life, individuals can support the yogic concept of prana, ensuring that their energy remains balanced and aligned. This holistic approach not only fosters inner peace but also upholds the ethical guidelines of yoga, promoting non-harm, compassion, and overall well-being.

Self-Awareness: Begin by cultivating self-awareness and understanding your energy levels, triggers, and boundaries. Reflect on past experiences where your energy may have been depleted or compromised due to a lack of boundaries.

Identify Your Boundaries: Take inventory of your physical, emotional, mental, and energetic boundaries. Determine what behaviors, situations, or interactions drain your energy or cause discomfort.

Communicate Your Boundaries Clearly: Practice assertive communication by clearly expressing your boundaries to others. Use "I" statements to convey your needs and preferences without blaming or shaming others. Be direct, specific, and respectful when communicating your boundaries.

Set Limits and Say No: Learn to set limits and say no to requests, commitments, or situations that do not align with your boundaries or priorities. Trust your instincts and intuition when determining whether to accept or decline invitations or obligations.

Protect Your Energy: Take proactive steps to protect your energy and prevent energetic drains or intrusions. Create physical, emotional, and energetic barriers when necessary to shield yourself from negative influences or excessive demands.

Practice Self-Care: Prioritize self-care practices that replenish and nourish your energy reserves. Dedicate daily time to activities that promote relaxation, rejuvenation, and inner peace, such as meditation, mindfulness, or time in nature.

Establish Healthy Relationships: Surround yourself with supportive individuals who respect and honor your boundaries. Set boundaries with toxic or energy-draining relationships, and consider minimizing or ending contact with individuals who consistently disregard your boundaries.

Regularly Reassess and Adjust: Regularly reassess your boundaries and evaluate whether they still serve your highest good. Be willing to adjust or renegotiate boundaries based on changes in circumstances, relationships, or personal growth. By establishing clear boundaries and prioritizing energetic balance, individuals can create a foundation for greater well-being, resilience, and empowerment. Remember that setting boundaries is an ongoing practice that requires self-awareness, assertiveness, and self-compassion.

Approach for Establishing Boundaries to Maintain Energetic Balance

Practice Grounding Techniques: Incorporate grounding techniques into your daily routine to anchor yourself in the present moment and maintain a strong connection with the Earth's energy. Techniques such as deep breathing, visualization, or walking barefoot in nature can help you feel centered and grounded, enhancing your ability to establish and maintain boundaries.

Use Visualization and Energetic Protection: Visualize yourself surrounded by a protective bubble of light or energy that acts as a barrier against negativity or unwanted influences. Practice energetic protection techniques, such as aura cleansing or shielding, to reinforce your boundaries and safeguard your energetic space.

Set Digital Boundaries: Establish boundaries around digital devices and online interactions to prevent energy drain and overwhelm. Schedule designated times for checking emails, social media, or messages, and turn off notifications outside of these times to minimize distractions and maintain focus.

Seek Support and Guidance: Contact trusted friends, family members, or mentors for support and guidance as you establish boundaries. Consider seeking the assistance of a coach, therapist, counselor, or energy healer who can provide additional insights and tools for maintaining energetic balance.

Practice Self-Compassion: Be gentle with yourself as you set and enforce boundaries, recognizing that it is a skill that takes time and practice to develop. Acknowledge any resistance or discomfort when asserting your boundaries, and remind yourself that prioritizing your well-being is essential for maintaining energetic balance.

Celebrate Progress and Successes: Celebrate your successes and milestones as you establish and maintain boundaries that support your energetic balance. Take time to acknowledge and appreciate the positive changes in your life due to honoring your boundaries and prioritizing your well-being.

Outcomes: By establishing boundaries, individuals can deepen their practice of maintaining energetic balance and creating a more supportive and nourishing environment for themselves. Remember that establishing boundaries is a dynamic process that evolves, and it is essential to remain flexible and adaptable as you navigate this journey of self-discovery and empowerment.

An Example of Establishing Boundaries to Maintain Energetic Balance in the Workplace

Scenario: Trevor is a software engineer working at a fast-paced tech company. He loves his job but often feels drained and overwhelmed by the demands of his workload and the pressure to always be available. Trevor realizes that he needs to establish boundaries to maintain his energetic balance and prevent burnout.

Self-Awareness: Trevor reflects on his exhaustion and stress, recognizing that his lack of boundaries contributes to his low energy levels and dissatisfaction with work.

Identify Your Boundaries: Trevor identifies his boundaries around work hours, communication expectations, and personal time. He realizes that he must limit how much time and energy he devotes to work daily.

Communicate Your Boundaries Clearly: Trevor communicates his boundaries to his manager and colleagues, explaining that he will set specific work hours and limit his availability outside those times. He uses assertive and respectful language to convey his needs and preferences, emphasizing the importance of work-life balance for his well-being.

Set Limits and Say No: Trevor learns to set limits on his workload and prioritize tasks based on urgency and importance. He practices saying no to additional projects or responsibilities that would exceed his capacity or compromise his boundaries.

Practice Self-Care: Trevor prioritizes self-care practices to replenish his energy and reduce stress. He schedules regular breaks throughout the day to rest, recharge, and engage in activities that bring him joy and relaxation. He also incorporates mindfulness and meditation into his routine to help him stay centered and grounded amidst work demands.

Establish Healthy Relationships: Trevor sets boundaries with his colleagues and clients to prevent work encroaching on his time. He communicates his availability and response times clearly and respectfully, setting expectations for communication outside of work hours. He nurtures his relationships with friends and family by setting aside dedicated time for social activities and quality time together, prioritizing connection and support outside work.

Regularly Reassess and Adjust: Trevor regularly reassesses his boundaries and evaluates their effectiveness in maintaining his energetic balance. He adjusts his boundaries as needed based on changes in workload, priorities, or personal circumstances. He remains flexible and adaptable, recognizing that establishing boundaries is an ongoing process that requires self-awareness and self-compassion.

By following this step-by-step approach, Trevor successfully establishes boundaries to maintain his energetic balance and prevent burnout in the workplace. He creates a healthier and more sustainable work-life balance that allows him to personally and professionally thrive.

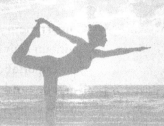

CHAPTER 22

Setting Boundaries While Starting New Relationships

Establishing boundaries in new relationships is crucial to ensure healthy interactions and mutual respect. Whether entering a romantic relationship, forming new friendships, or starting a new job, transparent and respectful boundaries help set expectations and protect your well-being. Integrating the principles of the eight limbs of yoga and Reiki can provide a holistic approach to boundary-setting.

Practical Steps for Setting Boundaries in New Relationships

1. **Self-Awareness (Svadhyaya & Reiki Self-Reflection):** Understand your needs, limits, and values before communicating them to others.

2. **Clear Communication (Satya & Reiki Honesty):** Be honest and straightforward when expressing your boundaries. Use "I" statements to take ownership of your needs.

3. **Consistency (Tapas & Reiki Discipline):** Maintain your boundaries consistently to reinforce their importance and ensure they are respected.

4. **Respect and Empathy (Ahimsa & Reiki Compassion):** Approach boundary-setting with compassion and understanding. Acknowledge the other person's perspective and needs as well.

5. **Moderation (Brahmacharya):** Balance your social interactions with personal commitments to avoid overextending yourself.

Setting Boundaries While Dating

Starting a new romantic relationship can be exciting, but it's crucial to establish boundaries early to ensure both partners feel respected and understood.

Scenario: Lance has started dating someone new. They've had a few dates, and things are going well. However, Lance values his personal space and needs time alone to recharge. He decides to communicate this early to avoid potential misunderstandings. During their third date, Lance shares, "I enjoy spending time with you, but I also value my time to recharge. I hope you understand that sometimes I need evenings to myself." This open and honest communication helps both partners respect each other's needs and establishes a foundation of mutual understanding.

Yogic Principle, Yama (Satya - Truthfulness): By speaking his truth with clarity and honesty, Lance ensures that his needs are understood and respected, fostering a healthy foundation for his relationship.

Reiki Principle, "Just for today, I will be honest and show gratitude for my many blessings": Lance's approach reflects honesty and gratitude, honoring the importance of clear communication in nurturing a respectful relationship.

Setting Boundaries with Friends

Forming new friendships involves understanding each other's comfort zones and respecting them.

Scenario: Monique has recently moved to a new city and is making new friends. She enjoys socializing but sometimes needs quiet time to unwind. Monique feels it might be too much for her when her new friend Leanne suggests a weekend-long getaway. She decides to set a boundary early in their friendship to avoid burnout. Monique tells Leanne, "I love hanging out with you, but I also need some downtime to relax. How about we plan to meet up on Saturday afternoon, and I'll keep Sunday for myself?" By expressing her needs, Monique ensures that her new friendship respects her limits.

Yogic Principle, Niyama (Svadhyaya - Self-Study): Monique's self-awareness allows her to recognize her need for rest and communicate it effectively, ensuring her well-being while forming new friendships.

Reiki Principle, "Just for today, I will honor all living creators": Monique honors her inner teacher by acknowledging her need for downtime and expressing it clearly.

Setting Boundaries with New Coworkers

Starting a new job comes with the challenge of establishing professional boundaries while building rapport with colleagues.

Scenario: Harvey has just started a job in the food service industry. He wants to be friendly with his coworkers but also maintains professionalism. Harvey is invited to join a casual after-work gathering on his first day. While he appreciates the gesture, he feels setting boundaries about his availability is essential. He politely declines by saying, "Thank you for the invitation! I'm still settling in and have some personal commitments tonight. Maybe next time?" This response helps Harvey set a clear boundary about his availability without appearing unfriendly.

Yogic Principle, Yama (Brahmacharya - Moderation): Harvey practices moderation by balancing his social life and personal commitments, ensuring he doesn't overcommit and overextend himself. Harvey's commitments could be anything from quiet time for himself to an important appointment. As long as it is important to Harvey and he committed it to himself it qualifies as a commitment.

Reiki Principle, "Just for today, I will not worry": Harvey's decision to set boundaries calmly and respectfully helps him avoid unnecessary stress and maintain a balanced work-life integration.

By implementing these steps and integrating the principles of yoga and Reiki, you can create healthy, respectful, and balanced new relationships. Whether dating, making friends, or starting a new job, clear boundaries ensure mutual respect and pave the way for positive interactions.

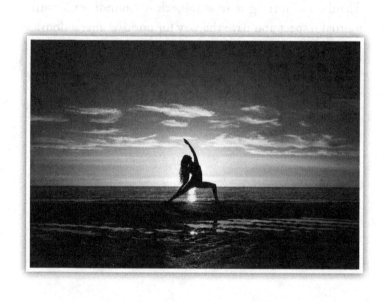

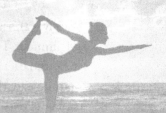

CHAPTER 23

Saying No with Compassion

Saying no is often challenging, as it can evoke feelings of guilt, fear of rejection, or concern about hurting others. However, setting boundaries is essential for maintaining our well-being and respecting our limits. The eight limbs of yoga and Reiki provide a supportive framework for saying no with compassion, ensuring our boundaries are communicated with kindness and clarity.

How the Eight Limbs of Yoga and Reiki Support Saying No with Compassion

1. **Yamas (Moral Restraints):** The Yamas guide us in our interactions with others, emphasizing non-violence (Ahimsa), truthfulness (Satya), and non-possessiveness (Aparigraha). Practicing these principles helps us to say no in a respectful and truthful way without causing harm.

2. **Niyamas (Personal Observances):** The Niyamas, including self-discipline (Tapas) and self-study

(Svadhyaya), encourage us to reflect on our needs and limits. This self-awareness enables us to set boundaries that honor our well-being and to communicate them.

3. **Asanas (Postures):** The physical practice of yoga postures helps to build strength and resilience, both physically and mentally. This resilience supports us in standing firm in our boundaries.

4. **Pranayama (Breath Control):** Pranayama practices help us to stay calm and centered, even in challenging situations. Deep, conscious breathing allows us to respond thoughtfully rather than react impulsively.

5. **Pratyahara (Withdrawal of the Senses):** Pratyahara encourages us to turn inward and tune out external distractions. This inward focus helps us to recognize when our boundaries are being compromised and to take action to protect them.

6. **Dharana (Concentration):** The practice of Dharana enhances our ability to concentrate and maintain focus on our priorities, making it easier to say no to distractions and unnecessary commitments.

7. **Dhyana (Meditation):** Meditation cultivates inner peace and clarity, allowing us to communicate our boundaries from a place of calmness and compassion.

8. **Samadhi (Union):** Achieving a state of Samadhi fosters a sense of oneness and interconnectedness. This awareness helps us understand that setting

boundaries is not about separation but maintaining harmony and balance.

Reiki's Role in Saying No with Compassion

Reiki energy work aligns with the principles of the eight limbs of yoga, promoting balance, harmony, and self-awareness. Reiki helps us to maintain an energetic balance, enabling us to set boundaries without feeling depleted or overwhelmed. The practice of Reiki also encourages us to approach boundary-setting with compassion, both for ourselves and for others.

An Example of How to Approach Saying No with Compassion

Scenario: Sharlene is a dedicated professional, a loving friend, and a caring family member. She often finds herself overwhelmed by work demands, social commitments, and family responsibilities. To protect her peace, Sharlene decides to practice saying no with compassion, supported by the principles of yoga and Reiki.

Protecting Peace at Home

Sharlene's family often expects her to handle all household chores, leaving her with little time for herself. She recognizes the need to set boundaries to maintain her well-being.

Self-Awareness (Svadhyaya): Sharlene reflects on her needs and realizes she requires time for self-care and relaxation.

Clear Communication (Satya): She communicates with her family, explaining her need for personal time and asking for their support in sharing household responsibilities.

Non-Attachment (Aparigraha): Sharlene lets go of the guilt associated with saying no to her family, understanding that her well-being is crucial for her to be present and supportive.

Maintaining Balance with Friends

Sharlene's friends frequently invite her to social gatherings, but she feels exhausted and needs rest.

Compassion (Ahimsa): Sharlene practices non-violence by being kind to herself and recognizing her need for rest.

Setting Boundaries (Tapas): She politely declines invitations, explaining that she needs to recharge.

Meditation (Dhyana): Sharlene uses meditation to stay centered and focused on her well-being, allowing her to say no without feeling guilty.

Navigating Work Commitments

Sharlene's colleagues often rely on her at work to take on additional tasks, leading to burnout.

Breath Control (Pranayama): Sharlene practices deep breathing to stay calm and composed when given extra tasks.

Concentration (Dharana): She focuses on her priorities, politely declining additional tasks that would compromise her well-being.

Energetic Balance (Reiki): Sharlene uses Reiki to balance her energy, ensuring she can maintain her boundaries without feeling drained.

Saying no with compassion is an essential skill for maintaining healthy boundaries and protecting our well-being. Yoga and Reiki provide a comprehensive framework for developing this skill, promoting self-awareness, clear communication, and inner peace. By embracing these practices, we can set boundaries that honor our needs and foster harmonious relationships with others.

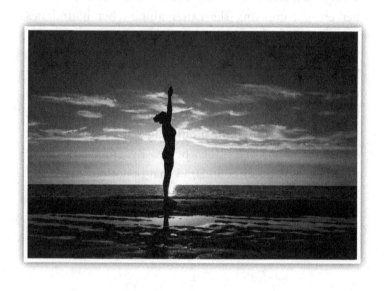

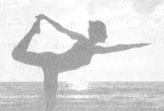

CHAPTER 24

Finding Balance in Boundaries

Setting boundaries is essential for maintaining emotional, mental, and physical well-being. However, it's common for people to overcorrect when they first start setting boundaries, leading to push back from others.

1. **Yama (Ethical Guidelines) & Reiki Ethics:**
   - **Ahimsa (Non-violence):** Set boundaries with kindness and compassion. Avoid being overly harsh or rigid.
   - **Satya (Truthfulness):** Communicate your boundaries honestly without aggression.
   - **Asteya (Non-stealing):** Respect others' time and energy as you set boundaries.
   - **Brahmacharya (Moderation):** Avoid extremes in your boundary-setting. Balance your needs with the needs of others.
   - **Aparigraha (Non-possessiveness):** Let go of the need to control others' reactions to your boundaries.

2. **Niyama (Personal Practices) & Reiki Self-care:**
    - **Saucha (Purity):** Keep your intentions clear and your communication clean.
    - **Santosha (Contentment):** Find peace in your decisions and respect others' boundaries.
    - **Tapas (Discipline):** Maintain consistency without being inflexible.
    - **Svadhyaya (Self-study):** Reflect on your needs and adjust boundaries as necessary.
    - **Ishvara Pranidhana (Surrender):** Trust the process and be open to change.

3. **Asanas (Postures) & Reiki Grounding:** Use physical postures to ground yourself and maintain personal space.

4. **Pranayama (Breath Control) & Reiki Energy Work:** Use breathwork to center yourself before communicating boundaries.

5. **Pratyahara (Withdrawal of Senses) & Reiki Sensitivity:** Develop awareness of your triggers and set boundaries to protect your energy.

6. **Dharana (Concentration) & Reiki Intent:** Focus on maintaining boundaries with clear intention.

7. **Dhyana (Meditation) & Reiki Mindfulness:** Regularly meditate on your boundaries and their effectiveness.

8. **Samadhi (Union) & Reiki Integration:** Strive for a harmonious balance in all your relationships.

Common Issues and Finding Balance

Overcorrection: When first establishing boundaries, it's easy to swing to extremes, becoming overly rigid or inflexible. This can create tension and pushback from others who may feel excluded or controlled.

Pushback from Others: People used to your old patterns may resist the new boundaries. They might test these boundaries or react negatively.

Reflect and Adjust (Svadhyaya & Reiki Self-Reflection): Regularly evaluate your boundaries. Are they too strict or too lenient? Adjust them based on what you learn about yourself and your interactions.

Communicate Compassionately (Ahimsa & Reiki Compassion): Explain your need for boundaries calmly and kindly. Understand that pushback is natural and approach it with empathy.

Stay Consistent (Tapas & Reiki Discipline): While flexible, ensure your boundaries are respected over time. Consistency helps others understand and adapt to your needs.

Practice Moderation (Brahmacharya): Balance your needs with others. Ensure your boundaries do not isolate you or create unnecessary conflict.

An Example of Finding Balance in Boundary Setting

Scenario: Matthew has recently started a new job. He's been feeling overwhelmed with the demands of his career and the expectations from his family and friends. Matthew decides to set boundaries to protect his time and energy.

Overcorrection: Matthew initially becomes very rigid, refusing to take calls or meet anyone after work. This leaves his family and friends feeling neglected and needing clarification. His friends start complaining that Matthew is avoiding them, and his family feels he's becoming distant. Matthew reflects on his needs and the feedback he's received. He decides to set specific times for personal time and family/friends' time. He communicates these new boundaries clearly and compassionately, explaining his need for balance and self-care.

By integrating the eight limbs of yoga and Reiki principles, Matthew can set healthy boundaries without alienating those he cares about. He learns to protect his energy while still being present for his loved ones, achieving a balanced approach to boundary-setting.

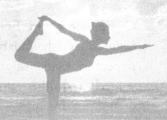

CHAPTER 25

A Recap of Key Concepts

Let's recap the key concepts and practices for setting healthy boundaries using the combined approaches of yoga and Reiki.

Self-Awareness and Mindfulness: Recognizing your needs, values, and limits is essential for setting healthy boundaries. Cultivating mindfulness through yoga and Reiki practices helps you stay present and attuned to your inner guidance.

Clarity and Communication: Communicating your boundaries assertively and respectfully is crucial in maintaining healthy relationships. Reiki intention and visualization techniques can reinforce your communication efforts and ensure your boundaries are understood.

Consistency and Self-Care: Maintaining your boundaries consistently over time requires dedication and self-discipline. Prioritizing self-care through practices like Reiki self-treatments and yoga helps you replenish your energy and uphold your boundaries effectively.

Compassion and Empathy: Balancing firmness with compassion in boundary setting fosters understanding and respect in relationships. Cultivating compassion towards yourself and others through Reiki compassion practices promotes harmonious interactions and mutual support.

Connection and Union: Understanding that healthy boundaries foster deeper connections and unity with others enhances the quality of your relationships. Recognizing the interconnectedness of all beings, as emphasized in yoga and Reiki teachings, encourages you to set boundaries that honor both your individuality and your connection to others.

Adaptability and Growth: Remaining open to adapting your boundaries as needed allows for personal growth and evolution. Reflecting on your boundary-setting practices regularly and integrating insights gained from yoga and Reiki practices supports your ongoing development and well-being.

By incorporating these key concepts and practices into your life, you can establish and maintain healthy boundaries that honor your needs, promote mutual respect, and foster greater harmony and balance in your relationships and overall well-being.

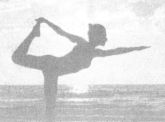

CHAPTER 26

Step by Step Approach to Setting Boundaries

Step 1: Self-Reflection and Awareness (Svadhyaya, Dhyana, and Reiki Self-Treatment)

Cultivate self-awareness through Svadhyaya (self-study) and Dhyana (meditation). Use Reiki self-treatment or alternate clearing mediation to clear any blockages and enhance self-awareness. Acknowledge areas where you may neglect your well-being due to a lack of boundaries. Recognize the impact of boundary violations on your physical, emotional, and spiritual health. Engage in journaling, meditation, or Reiki self-treatment to explore your emotions, triggers, and underlying beliefs.

Step 2: Clarify Your Boundaries (Satya, Dharana, and Reiki Ethics)

Identify specific areas where you need to establish boundaries. Use Dharana (concentration) to focus on what behaviors, actions, or situations cross your boundaries.

Define clear, specific boundaries that align with your values and priorities, grounded in Satya (truthfulness). Meditate on your boundaries, using Dharana to bring clarity and focus. Incorporate Reiki principles to maintain ethical and compassionate communication.

Step 3: Communicate Boundaries Clearly (Ahimsa, Satya, and Reiki Precepts)

Choose an appropriate time and place to communicate your boundaries. Express yourself honestly and directly, using "I" statements to communicate your feelings and needs. Practice Ahimsa (non-harm) and Satya (truthfulness) in setting and communicating your boundaries. Use compassionate communication, grounded in Reiki precepts, to express your boundaries with empathy and respect.

Step 4: Set Consequences (Asteya, Aparigraha, and Reiki Principles)

Communicate the consequences of boundary violations, if appropriate. Ensure the consequences are reasonable, proportionate, and enforceable. Uphold Asteya (non-stealing) by ensuring that your energy, time, and resources are not unfairly taken or depleted, and practice Aparigraha (non-attachment) by releasing the need to control others' reactions. Follow through with consequences consistently, supported by Reiki's ethical principles.

Step 5: Practice Self-Compassion (Santosha, Pratyahara, and Reiki Self-Care)

Be gentle with yourself as you navigate setting boundaries. Cultivate Santosha (contentment) by allowing yourself to prioritize your well-being. Use Pratyahara (withdrawal of senses) to focus inward, disconnecting from external pressures or expectations. Engage in Reiki self-care practices and Pratyahara techniques to nurture your physical, emotional, and spiritual well-being.

Step 6: Maintain Consistency (Tapas, Pranayama, and Reiki Discipline)

Stay committed to upholding your boundaries, even when it's challenging. Practice Tapas (discipline) and Pranayama (breath control) to reinforce your commitment. Use Pranayama to manage stress and maintain focus on your boundary-setting efforts. Integrate Reiki, meditation, and/ or affirmations into your routine, and practice Pranayama to enhance your discipline and consistency.

Step 7: Seek Support If Needed (Ishvara Pranidhana, Community, and other Support)

Contact trusted friends, family members, or professionals for support and guidance. Share your experiences and challenges with setting boundaries. Surrender to Ishvara Pranidhana (surrender to a higher power) and trust in the support of your community. Consider seeking the assistance of a coach, therapist, counselor, or energy healer. Yoga, Reiki, meditation individually and in group sessions to connect with supportive energy and guidance, surrendering to the divine flow of energy.

Step 8: Practice Self-Care (Saucha and Reiki Purification)

Prioritize self-care practices that nurture your well-being. Maintain Saucha (cleanliness) in your environment and energy field. Ensure your space and energy are clear and aligned with your boundaries. Engage in Reiki purification techniques and regular self-care rituals to keep your energy balanced and harmonious.

Step 9: Reflect and Adjust (Svadhyaya, Dhyana, and Meditation)

Regularly reflect on your boundary-setting process and its impact on your life. Use Dhyana (meditation) to deepen your reflection. Be open to learning and growing from your experiences, and be willing to adjust your boundaries as needed, supported by Svadhyaya (self-study). Use meditation to gain insight and make necessary adjustments to your boundaries.

Step 10: Embrace Unity and Wholeness (Samadhi and Reiki Oneness)

After reflecting on your boundary-setting journey and making necessary adjustments, embrace the sense of unity and wholeness that comes from living in alignment with your true self. Practice Samadhi to deepen your connection with the divine, achieving a state of oneness and inner peace.

Experience the profound sense of connection and harmony that comes from setting boundaries that honor your authentic self. Recognize that boundaries are not just about separation but also about creating a sacred space for your true essence to thrive.

Engage in deep meditation to enter a state of Samadhi, where the boundaries between self and the universe dissolve. Use Reiki to enhance this state of oneness, allowing the universal life force to flow freely within you, affirming your interconnectedness with all things.

Outcome: This holistic, step-by-step approach allows you to set boundaries that honor your truth, prioritize your well-being, and foster healthy relationships. Integrating all Eight Limbs of Yoga with Reiki principles creates a balanced and comprehensive framework for living authentically and respecting yourself and others. This plan promotes personal growth, well-being, and spiritual alignment, guiding you toward a more empowered and harmonious life.

In the context of boundary-setting, Samadhi represents the culmination of your efforts. It's the realization that by setting and respecting boundaries, you create a foundation for spiritual growth and inner peace. Boundaries allow you to maintain your individuality while also connecting deeply with others and the world around you. This state of unity, supported by the ethical and spiritual principles of Reiki, reflects the balance and harmony that boundaries bring to your life.

This integration of Samadhi reminds you that the ultimate goal of boundary-setting is not just to protect yourself but to live in harmony with your true self and the world around you, achieving a state of peace, wholeness, and spiritual enlightenment.

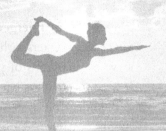

CHAPTER 27

A Message to Seekers of Boundaries and Balance

Dear Seeker of Boundaries and Balance,

As you journey on the path of self-discovery and growth, remember that setting healthy boundaries is not just a one-time task but an ongoing process of self-care and empowerment. Each step you take towards establishing and maintaining boundaries that honor your well-being is a courageous act of self-love and respect.

Embrace Your Evolution: Acknowledge and celebrate how far you've come in your boundary-setting journey. Every boundary you've set, every lesson you've learned, and every boundary you've honored has contributed to your growth and evolution. Embrace the process, knowing that each experience offers opportunities for deeper understanding and self-awareness.

Nourish Your Energetic Balance: Just as the chakras are vital energy centers within your subtle body, your boundaries serve as guardians of your energetic balance. Explore the interconnectedness between your chakras, energy system, and endocrine system, understanding how imbalances in one area can impact the others. By nurturing your chakras through practices like yoga, Reiki, and meditation, you support the flow of energy throughout your being, promoting harmony and vitality.

Continued Education and Exploration: Stay curious and open to learning more about boundary-setting chakras and energy anatomy. Dive deeper into the wisdom of ancient teachings and modern modalities, seeking knowledge that resonates with your journey. Explore how each chakra corresponds to specific aspects of your physical, emotional, and spiritual well-being and how you can harness this knowledge to support your boundary-setting efforts.

Empowerment Through Awareness: Remember that awareness is vital to empowerment. Tune into your body, mind, and spirit, listening to the whispers of your intuition and the guidance of your inner wisdom. Trust yourself to know what boundaries serve your highest good and have the courage to honor them, even when it's challenging.

Support and Connection: You are not alone on this journey. Seek support from trusted friends, mentors, or professionals who can offer guidance and encouragement along the way. Share your experiences, insights, and challenges with others who understand and respect your path.

Infinite Potential: Know that you possess endless potential within you. As you continue to grow and evolve in your boundary-setting journey, embrace the limitless possibilities that await you. Trust in your innate strength, resilience, and capacity for transformation.

May you walk your path with confidence, grace, and authenticity, knowing that you are worthy of setting boundaries that honor your truth and support your well-being. May you find empowerment, balance, and joy in every step of your journey.

With love and light,
Harmony

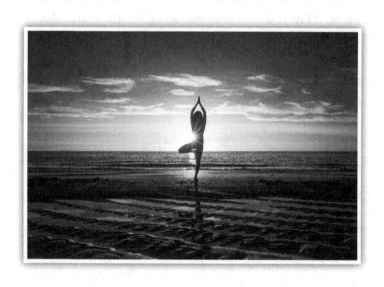

ABOUT THE AUTHOR

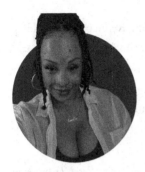

Lenise "Harmony" Halley is a multifaceted wellness expert with a deep foundation in health and personal development. As a Professional Certified Coach (ICF-PCC), a National Academy of Sports Medicine Certified Personal Trainer (NASM-CPT), a Usui/Holy Fire® III Reiki Master Teacher, and an experienced Yoga Teacher (E-RYT® 500, YACEP®), Harmony integrates mind, body, and spiritual wellness into a holistic approach for personal growth.

Her clients are empowered to reach their healthiest, most balanced selves through practices that nurture the mind, body, and soul, all while embracing the joy of play. Inspired by her transformative journey, Harmony provides practical self-exploration exercises, helping clients uncover their deepest desires and equipping them with tools to achieve a life of wealth, wellness, and harmony.

Visit GotHarmony.org for more resources.

Books by Harmony- *Got Harmony?: Quick Guide to Living Your Best Life* — A practical guide offering actionable steps for a balanced, fulfilling life.

Online Courses and Coaching- Explore boundary-setting, yoga philosophy, and Reiki energy work with personalized coaching and online courses.

In-Person Yoga Classes- Join supportive yoga classes at various locations to deepen your practice, cultivate mindfulness, and explore yoga philosophy.

Community and Events- Connect with like-minded individuals through Harmony's events, workshops, and retreats. Follow on social media or subscribe to the blog for updates.

BIBLIOGRAPHY

"5 Essential Measures to Manage and Reduce Stress." Help Health. https://www.helphealth.co/2021/07/stress-5-measures.html

Arnsten, Amy F.T. "Stress Signalling Pathways that Impair Prefrontal Cortex Structure and Function." Nature Reviews Neuroscience, vol. 10, no. 6, 2009, pp. 410-422. doi:10.1038/nrn2648.

Brown, Brene. *Rising Strong: How the Ability to Reset Transforms the Way We Live, Love, Parent, and Lead.* Spiegel & Grau, 2015.

Chopra, Deepak. *The Book of Secrets: Unlocking the Hidden Dimensions of Your Life.* Harmony Books, 2004.

Emerson, David. *Trauma-Sensitive Yoga in Therapy: Bringing the Body into Treatment.* W. W. Norton & Company, 2015.

Iyengar, B.K.S. *Light on Life: The Yoga Journey to Wholeness, Inner Peace, and Ultimate Freedom.* Rodale, 2005.

Judith, Anodea. *Eastern Body, Western Mind: Psychology and the Chakra System as a Path to the Self.* Celestial Arts, 2004.

Kabat-Zinn, Jon. *Full Catastrophe Living: Using the Wisdom of Your Body and Mind to Face Stress, Pain, and Illness.* Bantam Dell, 1990.

Kabat-Zinn, Jon. *Wherever You Go, There You Are: Mindfulness Meditation in Everyday Life.* Hyperion, 1994.

LeDoux, Joseph E. "Emotion Circuits in the Brain." Annual Review of Neuroscience, vol. 23, no. 1, 2000, pp. 155-184. doi:10.1146/annurev.neuro.23.1.155.

McTaggart, Lynne. *The Field: The Quest for the Secret Force of the Universe*. Harper Perennial, 2008.

Motoyama, Hiroshi. *Theories of the Chakras: Bridge to Higher Consciousness*. Quest Books, 1981.

Patanjali. *The Yoga Sutra of Patanjali*. Translated by Sri Swami Satchidananda, Integral Yoga Publications, 2012.

Rand, William Lee. *Reiki for Dummies*. For Dummies, 2005.

Rand, William Lee. *Reiki: The Healing Touch*. Vision Publications, 1991

Reiki, William Lee. T*he Healing Art of Reiki: A Beginner's Guide*. CreateSpace Independent Publishing Platform, 2017.

Sapolsky, Robert M. *Why Zebras Don't Get Ulcers: The Acclaimed Guide to Stress, Stress-Related Diseases, and Coping*. 3rd ed., Henry Holt and Co., 2004.

Stein, Diane. *Essential Reiki: A Complete Guide to an Ancient Healing Art*. Crossing Press, 1995.

Swami Sivananda. *The Science of Pranayama*. The Divine Life Society, 1998.

Tiwari, Swami. *The Path of Yoga: An Essential Guide to Its Principles and Practices*. Shambhala Publications, 2002.

Tolle, Eckhart. *The Power of Now: A Guide to Spiritual Enlightenment*. New World Library, 1999.

van der Kolk, Bessel A. *The Body Keeps the Score: Brain, Mind, and Body in the Healing of Trauma*. Penguin Books, 2015.

Williamson, Marianne. *A Return to Love: Reflections on the Principles of "A Course in Miracles."* HarperCollins, 1992.

Printed in the United States
by Baker & Taylor Publisher Services